I'm Still Standing

My Fight Against Hereditary Breast Cancer

WENDY WATSON

**SIMON &
SCHUSTER**

London · New York · Sydney · Toronto · New Delhi

A CBS COMPANY

First published in Great Britain by Simon & Schuster UK Ltd, 2011
A CBS Company

1 3 5 7 9 10 8 6 4 2

Simon & Schuster UK Ltd
1st Floor
222 Gray's Inn Road
London
WC1X 8HB

www.simonandschuster.co.uk

Simon & Schuster Australia,
Sydney

Simon & Schuster India, New Delhi

A CIP catalogue for this book is available
from the British Library.

ISBN: 978-0-85720-846-0
Typeset by Hewer Text UK Ltd, Edinburgh
Printed and bound by CPI Group (UK) Ltd, Croydon, CR0 4YY

To all my family and friends who have supported me throughout the years. To the wonderful volunteers who have given tirelessly, and to local sponsors without whose help survival would have been impossible – in particular Professor Gareth Evans, who has been my constant friend, supporter and advisor throughout.

Heartfelt and grateful thanks to Becky for nominating me as Mum of the Year, and Garry Blackman and Tesco for their invaluable help in finding a suitable high-profile publisher. Thanks to Angela Herlihy, my editor, and for additional editorial input from John Squires and Mary Marshall.

Lastly many thanks to Anne De Waal for inspiring me to write the book in the first place.

Contents

A Few Words from Linda Robson

I first heard about the wonderful Wendy Watson when I was asked to be on the judging panel of the Tesco Magazine Mum of the Year Awards in 2011. Myself and the other judges were sent each mum's profile and, although all of them were impressive women in their own ways, Wendy stood out for us. We came to a unanimous decision and voted her Overall Mum of the Year.

As women and mothers, we just could not get over how Wendy and her daughter Becky had made their life-changing decisions to have preventative mastectomies at such young ages. It seemed unimaginable to me. And how traumatic must it have been to take the genetic test and find out that Wendy had the faulty gene, but her sister Diane did not. Life is such at lottery at times. A couple of my close friends have suffered with breast cancer so I know the horror of the disease.

At the awards ceremony, I met Wendy and her lovely family – Becky, her sister Diane and their father, who seemed so proud of his daughter. I was knocked out by how warm and open Wendy was, and how her positive attitude must have helped many others when they have turned to her for help. Not only did she choose to live, but she decided not to wallow in her own situation and reached out to other people to help them. She really is an inspiration and a fantastic person.

Linda Robson, July 2011

Foreword
by Professor Gareth Evans

Wendy Watson is a remarkable woman. I first met her in 1992 when, to escape her appalling family history of breast cancer, she had decided her only logical option was to undergo a risk-reducing double mastectomy. Two months later, removal of her ovaries to prevent ovarian cancer lifted the fear of the disease from her.

After Wendy was involved in the Channel 4 documentary *Living in the Shadow* in 1994 with me and the rest of her family, she began being approached by other women concerned about their risks. When Wendy was pivotal in two sisters getting their referral to discuss risk-reducing mastectomies, she realised what a powerful advocate she could be. We travelled down to London together to discuss hereditary breast cancer with the then Health Minister, Baroness Cumberlege, who suggested setting up a helpline and offered a small amount of government funding. Set Wendy any task and she will strive to achieve it. That is why she is such an amazing advocate for patients.

The rest is history. Wendy has provided a magnificent service to patients, always knowing when to temper pathos with humour. She never pushes women into making decisions they don't want, but guides and supports them in making the best individual decisions for themselves. She has received literally thousands of calls, sometimes in the middle of the night! Battles are nothing new to Wendy. Fighting for the survival of the helpline would continue to her dying breath. She has fought the might of government opinion to oppose the European patent directive that made it legal to patent genes. Now the UK and other European governments realise the mistake in allowing such generic patents.

As part of the NICE guideline development group for familial breast cancer, Wendy has been vital in opinion-forming. She lectures all round the UK and has been to Europe and America to talk about the helpline. She will not pass up an opportunity to get the message out there about hereditary breast cancer.

Please do not think this book is all about struggle and gloom. Wendy injects wonderful humour into everything and is a great raconteur. Her story is one of success in persuading the medical profession, politicians and the press to support her amazing cause.

Professor D Gareth Evans MD FRCP
Consultant in Genetic Medicine

Prologue

Eight nervous mums line up outside the Palm Court room, ready to parade in to the music, just as we had done several times earlier in rehearsal. The music starts, the door is opened, and as I proudly lead everyone on, remembering to stop in a line at the top of the stairs, I take in the opulent splendour of it all. I can only marvel that this lavish event, honouring the chosen mums, could include ordinary me.

Looking around at the tables crowded with celebrities, friends, families, directors of Tesco, and the whole team who put this huge event together, every one of them clapping, cheering and warmly effusive in their welcome, I am suddenly hit with the idea that 'ordinary me' has indeed led anything but an ordinary life. In fact, the most extraordinary chain of events has led to this award.

I take my allocated seat, next to the lovely bubbly Linda Robson, and the lavish, perfectly served lunch leads into the awards ceremony. The short film that *Tesco Magazine* has made about me sums things up beautifully.

It explains how I decided that the only way to protect myself from developing the breast cancer that was so rife in my family was to have a double mastectomy *before* the cancer occurred. I've subsequently battled to help the world see this as a reasonable course of action for those with a genetic predisposition to the disease, and to educate everyone about *all* the options available. There were so many hurdles to deal with en route that could never have been envisaged. I wanted choice for people so they could make their own decisions about their own lives and, in the film, internationally renowned Consultant Geneticist, Professor Gareth Evans, credits me with having done just that. He states that I changed for the better the way the medical profession viewed hereditary breast cancer. Clips are shown of me having to take on the European Parliament, challenging multi-million pound lobbies. How could I ever have imagined that? But equally, I could never have imagined being here in front of all these people, with celebrities standing to applaud. Within those four minutes, people have both laughed out loud and also cried.

Hostess and presenter Fiona Phillips asks me about aspects of my story, and Emilia Fox presents me with the award of Overall Winner, Mum of the Year, saying how remarkable everything is that has been achieved. But no – it's just how it happened. What I did simply had to be done – not only to find a way to stay alive myself, but to help others in a similar position. I had no idea at the outset that this journey would take so many twists and turns.

The rollercoaster ride that is my life, the surreal situations that have befallen me, are a constant fascination to many: running a 24-hour helpline every day, training 22 others with little or no funding.

However, very few other things in life have presented me with a fear that I couldn't conquer. To me, most things can be tackled head on. Objections to causes I strongly believe in? I have just viewed these as obstacles to be overcome; removed or kicked down if necessary in order to make life work. It is always easy to fight something you feel justifiably passionate about.

And that just about sums up my life: laughing and fighting. It helps if you can see the funny side to all the silly situations you are asked to deal with. My own sense of humour has stood me in good stead over the years. Giggling is still a problem for me at times, although I thought I would grow out of it by now, at the age of 55! Yes, to quote Sir Elton John, 'I'm Still Standing'!

Why tell my story now? As good a time as any, I guess.

So, here goes.

BEGINNINGS

I was born in Derby City Hospital in January 1955 to Stewart and Jean Watson; their first child. Five months later Mum and Dad moved into a bungalow in Breaston, a small village between Nottingham and Derby. The surrounding area was unremarkable. Very flat, with neither huge wealth nor dire poverty, it was just an ordinary growing village with a church, a chapel and about a dozen shops. My earliest memories are of Diane, my sister, who arrived when I was four. I remember going to hospital to fetch Mum back home. I hadn't seen my sister at this point because I don't think children were allowed in hospitals, so I sat in the back of the car with Aunty Kath, waiting to inspect this new addition. I remember saying, 'I can't stop my face from smiling' – a phrase that the adults repeated regularly as they obviously found it cute.

My first exposure to fame in the media was evidently in a similar vein. I used to love helping Mum with the baking and once I asked, at the point of brushing the milk onto the cake with the pastry brush, 'Mummy, please may I sweep the cake?' unwittingly earning

Mum ten shillings because she wrote to the letters page of *Woman* magazine and was paid for publishing it. Ah, the innocence! Such wonderful days and worth reminiscing over. I'm sure my mother wouldn't have been the only one to swallow a toddler's overfilled jam tart, its pastry grey, and rapturously declare how delicious it was.

I would settle down to *Watch with Mother* with Diane, and on Andy Pandy days (Tuesdays, for those with short memories) I would place a cardboard box on our settee to replicate the picnic hamper that he and Teddy hopped into at the end of each episode. We went through the entire ritual of singing 'Andy Pandy's coming to play, tra, la la, la laa la', dancing with Louby Lou, and finishing with 'Andy is waving goodbye' as the hamper lid closed. Diane and I would squash into the cardboard box, imitating all the manoeuvres throughout the programme.

However, there were occasional 'gloomy Sundays', around four times a year, when we visited Great-Great Aunty Alice and Uncle Arthur in Lenton, on the outskirts of Nottingham. Yes, my grandfather's elderly aunty and uncle. I say gloomy because, whatever the weather, their Victorian bay-windowed, semidetached house would always cast a deep depression over me. It was terrifying. The front door opened into a dark, narrow passageway with a very high ceiling and an echoing floor. The front room to the left of this passage was no better. The fireplace was cast iron, under a dark, imposing mantelpiece. Just to complete the overbearing picture, in the bay window was a giant aspidistra, whose role was obviously to blank out any remaining sunlight that had managed to sneak past the overgrown privet hedge outside.

My principle aim on these visits was to refuse all drinks and thus reduce the need to brave the trip upstairs to the toilet. The few occasions I had to use it, I did so with bated breath, convinced that I would be overpowered by some ghoulish thing hiding in the darker shadows. How anyone could live there was beyond me. Great-Great Aunty Alice had a beard, which I just assumed came with living to 95.

After the predictable tea of ham sandwiches and cake, they would play a game of cards – Newmarket I think it was called – while I was given a jar of farthings to play with on the floor. To say I hated those occasions is a gross understatement. I think the visits stopped when I was still very young, as I guess our elderly relatives must have died. I can't pretend I wasn't thankful!

My paternal grandmother's home was the complete reverse. It was cosy, friendly and warm, and I loved visiting. Grandma Watson was the sweetest, kindliest lady ever. She had an enormous bosom, a truly mountainous affair, generally covered by a flowery apron. Little wonder that my father grew to be six-foot-four after being fed from these mammoth vessels! The only hazard of this visit was being sat on Nana's knee, trying to find a way to breathe whilst enduring a cuddle. I quickly learnt that it was important to wriggle slightly away to ensure that breathing was still a possibility. After Diane was born, I was relieved of this cuddle duty somewhat because baby Diane would lie quietly in this position. Maybe she was semi-comatose after being smothered, but she seemed to bear no lasting ill effects.

Other very early memories are my first day at school, meeting a girl who was to become my best friend. Our assignment was to draw something about Christmas, and Linda was an artist with Christmas trees. What Linda couldn't portray with a set of green triangles was nobody's business. Plus, she had the best set of pencils! We made great friends and remain so to this day.

Early school days were my introduction to the magical world of Enid Blyton. Our teacher, Mrs Mellors, would read us stories about the Magic Faraway Tree every Friday afternoon. Different clouds would arrive each week to the top of this tree, each one a new land. Some lands were exciting and nice like the Land of Sweets or the Land of Do As You Please. Others were dangerous and scary like the Land of Dame Slap's school. Whatever the land, I just loved the adventure and mystery.

My overactive imagination was easily fired by the various adventures and mysteries solved by the Famous Five, the Secret Seven, Five Find-Outers and Dog, and other such glorious Enid Blyton series. The excitement of their adventures filled me with the greatest enthusiasm for visiting old houses. (By this stage I had recovered from the horrors of Great-Great Aunty Alice's residence!) I always imagined this would be where I might find a secret panel, leading to a secret passage. I was also totally convinced that I would be the very first to discover it. Every panel would be tapped in all four corners, while I waited excitedly for the mechanism to spring into action and slide it to one side.

Linda and I started our own detective agency. We enthusiastically collected clues and suspects, just waiting for a mystery to come along to fit in with our ready detective work. Sadly, our suspects were never brought to task, they thoughtlessly never seemed to commit any crimes, and the clues lay unused in Linda's shed.

Little did I realise, however, just how much detective work I would be involved with in later life. Enid Blyton gave me a damned good grounding!

Unfortunately, I never did discover a secret passage, so I set about digging one of my own. Sadly, this came to a swift and sudden end when I soon hit water, which I realised would be an insurmountable problem. Childhood was a time for excitement and adventure. The village of Breaston was quiet, the roads weren't busy, especially our side roads. Building sites were springing up everywhere with early 1960s housing, and this gave rise to fabulous play areas. The heaps and tips of soil dug out and dumped created fantastic undulations for our cycle racecourse. My bike was my sturdy friend. I loved the fields and countryside; the homing ground for catching butterflies for the butterfly house I had built.

White mice suddenly became my next project when I was about eight years old. A new girl had arrived on the street, and she had two of them. I really fell for these cute little things, so I researched the cost and found a pet shop that charged one and sixpence per mouse. Mum and Dad clearly did not share my new passion so, with my savings and Christmas money, I amassed the grand total of three shillings; just enough to buy a breeding pair. Unfortunately, the plan was thwarted as I did not have enough money to purchase the mouse hutch. Mum and Dad didn't offer to assist here at all, and I'm sure they were convinced that this small obstacle would bring the end to this particular craze.

Not so! I scoured the garage for suitable pieces of wood, glue, a hammer, nails and, the pièce de résistance, floorboarding with magnificent grooves in which one could slide a piece of glass up and down. With Dad's best saw, I set to work on his workbench in the garage. Cutting the glass presented no problem for a child as resourceful as I was. Diamonds cut glass, didn't they? Mum's diamond engagement ring did the trick nicely – a bit jagged, but passable. The mice even had an upstairs floor with a staircase: a piece of wood with spent matches glued to it. I really was proud of this masterpiece.

So, reluctantly, Dad took me on Saturday morning to buy my pair of white mice. I was desperately excited, ready to choose Albert and Alice, my already named pets. The man in the pet shop asked if we wanted them to be of opposite sexes, of which I was adamantly in favour. Dad, meanwhile, was quietly signalling 'no' to the shop owner.

At home I spent hours tipping the poor mice on their backs trying to identify the sexes. Moving their tails side to side, backwards and forwards, in order to deduce some apparent difference, but to no avail. I couldn't detect anything at all, they seemed identical to me. It didn't matter anyway, as by Sunday morning the mice had eaten their way through a corner in the hardboard and escaped— never to be seen again!

After the mice and Enid Blyton, an eventful visit to see *Mary Poppins* at the cinema gave me the craze to learn to fly with an umbrella. The Mary Poppins era almost ended in disaster. We had a bungalow. Outside our bungalow there was a coke bunker, and Diane and I spent hours practising how to fly, umbrellas held high. After the first few failed attempts, I decided it was just a matter of logistics. The coke bunker just wasn't high enough, so plans were in place to get Diane onto the roof of the bungalow . . . Unfortunately she didn't fly from there either!

The next phase involved horses, which were destined to become an enduring passion (with a brief intermission for make-up, clothes and boys, but to return again later in life). My pocket money had risen to a massive four shillings per week by the time I was nine, which was exactly the price of a half-hour lesson at our local riding school. Now, this is an era I remember vividly and with nostalgia for the horsey smells, the camaraderie, the sheer joy of being on horseback and mastering the art of riding. My biggest ever thrill came from winning my first rosette at a local gymkhana. It was fourth place in the showing class, and I still have that little green rosette. I was so proud I could have burst.

Of course, this fired me with the desire to acquire my own horse, but it seemed a somewhat grander task than raising three shillings for a pair of mice. Their 'housing' seemed easier to overcome though. At the bottom of our garden was next door's orchard. I visited Mrs Woodcock, the owner, and asked if I might rent their orchard to graze a pony. I'm sure they thought the plans must have been further forward than they actually were. I was busy brokering a deal with my four shillings per week as rent. The more difficult solution was where to get the required fifty pounds to purchase a pony in the first place. The saddlery and rugs were an issue too. I reluctantly had to satisfy myself with the 'virtual' horses in my head, which were almost a reality to me. One I called Coffee, a beautiful liver chestnut with a flaxen mane and tail, and one called Jigsaw. Obviously a skewbald!

I satisfied myself with building a showjumping course in our garden. Every available plank of wood was painted red and white, or blue and white. Stands were made with nails sticking out on which to lodge these poles at different heights. 'Water jumps' were dug out in front of the rockery. One day, I returned from the dentist having had the day off school, and noticed a set of rustic poles propped up at the side of the bungalow. Excitement overcame me. By tea-time they were transformed into six beautiful red and white showjumping poles and neatly propped up in the garage, drying. I couldn't wait to proudly tell my generous dad that the poles he had ordered for me were stripped, painted, and ready for action. Amazingly, it didn't quite elicit the reaction of approval I was expecting. Dad appeared, selfishly, to have ordered these poles to make a rustic trellis. How silly. And what a tremendous waste! At least I put them to good use.

Diane occasionally succumbed to being tied round the waist with the washing line and obediently walking, trotting and cantering in circles around me, whilst I trained this new, young horse. I had to make a deal though, that the 'lunge whip' I had manufactured myself was cracked at a safe distance from her, otherwise she would sulk and go indoors. So boring when one's little sister stops co-operating!

We used to share other fun projects, though. Midnight feasts were a regular item on our agenda, rarely actually happening, but the plans were thrilling. Actually I learned a great deal about anticipation and planning as a child and acquired a particular piece of wisdom which is rarely acknowledged. The planning and anticipation of an event is often the best bit. The reality can be a disappointment, after all the vivid imaginings and speculation.

My sister and I shared a bedroom, our headquarters for planned mischief. Diane was always a very well-behaved child, looking to me to provide 'big sister' leadership in some of the scrapes and activities we got into. At the age of six, however, Diane surpassed even me in these scrapes. She had a stamp collection. She was a very keen collector – so keen that one day she faced threats of legal action from the Bridgenorth Stamp Club for stamps she had been sent on approval, but not paid for! I remember the threatening letter arriving. I have no idea how this was resolved, but I do know that she managed to escape a criminal record from the event.

Diane was, and still is, really pretty. I envied her prettiness, as I think she envied some of my daredevil courage, but we never displayed any jealousies towards each other. I took up my first job at the age of 10, a paper round. Diane was my first employee. At the tender age of six she would get up with me early on Friday mornings to help with the double load on *Long Eaton Advertiser* day. Everyone in Breaston seemed to take the *Advertiser* along with their usual daily paper, making for two loads and a halfway trip back to the newsagent's for the next bagful. I paid Diane a shilling per week for services rendered, but I'm afraid I always used to owe her several weeks of back pay. She soon became a little accountant in her own right. Often she was the only one in the house with any money – I think even Dad borrowed from her at times. However, she was astute. She devised a ledger in her special notebook, of monies owed to her. I'm not certain if I don't still owe about five shillings actually!

Those cold mornings on the paper round were comical. I would dress Diane up in her balaclava helmet. She had short hair with a fringe, and always slept face down. So, she always had a lovely tuft of hair sticking up at the front, earning her the nickname of Tufty, which she hated. She would mount her tricycle, which was very useful on Friday's paper round as it was equipped with a little boot. I gave her training on where to post each newspaper. I can still see in my mind's eye this little figure on the blue tricycle, peddling like fury up and down the driveways.

Mum was an excellent cook. She did all her own baking, as I'm sure all mums did in the early 1960s. Her meat and potato pie was legendary, and she was an excellent pastry chef, a talent certainly not passed on to me. Diane is the one who inherited these incredible talents, and is a superb cook and homemaker. Mum was a born homemaker too. She loved making jam, and our house would often have large pans bubbling away on the stove. She used to make the most delicious lemon drink when we had colds. Diane and I were really excited if we felt a cold coming on because we knew that several pounds of sugar and half a dozen lemons would soon be heating away in a large jug on the stove. Another memory of my mum – and they mostly seem to be connected with food – is raspberry vinegar. This is truly delicious. Mum would make extra Yorkshire puddings on Sundays, sometimes to have as dessert with this raspberry vinegar poured over them. We used to go on trips and outings to pick blackberries for my favourite blackberry and apple pie. In fact, Mum was, I'm sure, at her happiest in the kitchen.

She also worked as a schoolteacher, and threw herself into the village community, joining 'Young Wives' and other such groups. I remember a phase of hat-making at Young Wives when she had various strange-shaped bases upon which different materials were fastened. Dad came home one day with two wood pigeons he had shot, so I plucked them and attempted to make a hat for Mum using these feathers. I can't remember it being worn though!

Mum was definitely the coffee-morning type. We went on endless rounds of these events at various neighbours' houses and village halls. Mum taught me to play cards at a very young age, which I loved immensely. She swiftly taught me to play Patience, which allowed her to get on with housework. We would all attend whist drives and beetle drives as a family, Mum being one of the organisers. I spent many hours putting raffle tickets on tombola items for the many worthy causes Young Wives supported.

Times were not easy in those days, and Diane and I would have one new dress each year for the Sunday school anniversary. The remainder of our clothes Mum made for us. There was always some garment or other on the sewing machine. Having an industrious mother allowed me the space for my own explorations and endless reading.

One thing was guaranteed, though, that my enormous appetite as a child would be fully satisfied. Dinners were always bang on time and we were expected to be back and ready from whatever we had been up to. I guess I would have been rewarding to feed since I always used to declare at each meal, 'This was my very best favourite!'

Diane and I weren't too old before we realised that Santa Claus never came to either Mum or Dad, which seemed totally wrong in our eyes. We therefore hatched a brilliant plot to make amends here and resolve this particular injustice. We both had school plimsoll bags, so we set about visiting the church jumble sale and bazaar and buying items to wrap up lovingly and put in each home-made 'Santa sack' for our poor, hard-done-by parents. The joys of giving were soon discovered. That Christmas was just so thrilling; to find things we could afford in order to make lots of presents for our parents to open. I'm sure they brought all their acting skills to the fore on that Christmas morning as they unwrapped chipped china ashtrays, scarves, vases and other such valuable items. I really think they also genuinely shared some of our excitement.

I spent quite a considerable few years being a real 'horsey bore', as Dad put it. I felt a huge responsibility for looking after my two imaginary horses to the best of my ability. All 566 pages of *Summerhays' Encyclopaedia for Horsemen* were dutifully studied and absorbed. I have always had a photographic memory, which enables rote learning almost to the point of cheating. The success of my Eleven-plus exams and subsequent secondary school exams, was reliant totally on this photographic memory. The only things I really enjoyed at school, apart from games and gym of course, were maths (puzzles), English (books), drama (loved acting and singing) and languages (the exotic travels they conjured up in my imagination).

Linda and I discovered the joys of shopping for make-up and other girly accessories around the age of 13. Together, we were incorrigible gigglers. Trying on preposterous hats in our local department store was a firm favourite, only moving on after our squeals of laughter at each other elicited the stern disapproval of the elegant shop assistants. So different nowadays; those immaculately coiffured ladies were always ready to pounce, whereas now it seems impossible to find one in a large department store. Linda still adores shopping with a passion. I am not so keen.

We had just started to attend our local youth club,

but swiftly developed the urge to travel further afield, searching for more interesting boys. We were a group of four or five girlfriends, and the local youth club had only one fanciable boy who, unfortunately, was already dating a very pretty girl. Soon, we travelled every Friday night to Long Eaton, to the heady discotheque where thrilling 1960s music was played, and mods and rockers seemed to coexist fairly amicably in that neck of the woods. To this day I still love the Four Tops, and most of the Motown music.

It was a great privilege to be a teenager in the 1960s, coinciding with The Beatles, flower power, hippies, Motown, miniskirts, flares and hotpants. We learnt to prance around, showing off our super-slim waists, extra-long legs, and not-so-ample bosoms. Boyfriends came and went.

Linda's family would regularly take me on holiday with them as she was an only child. The Lake District was an annual event. Linda's father and I were the most intrepid and would tackle the more challenging climbs. I always wanted to climb everywhere just to see what was round the corner and exactly what was at the top. Linda was content on those occasions to sit by the tarns, companionably reading with her mother. I was always active and sporty and loved running and jumping.

In the Lake District we always stayed at a very homely B&B in Bassenthwaite. Now, for two girls whose minds were firmly occupied by clothes, make-up and boys, the nightlife was nonexistent, so Linda and I would spend hours getting ready for the evening meal. Full make-up was always essential although it was just ourselves, and maybe one other (usually elderly) couple resident in that small boarding house. I remember Linda's dad saying to us both, 'I don't know why you two want to spend so much time putting all this trifle on your eyes.' I suppose the colours may have been rather exotic, and perhaps a tad out of place amongst the hiking boots and rucksacks!

I was glad of these holidays with my pal. Dad had started a small printing business of his own, working in the evenings after finishing his day job at Rolls-Royce, and family holidays were not a high priority. We used to visit Abersoch, on the Llyn Penninsula in Wales, each year, and had various caravan holidays there which we all loved. But as my sister and I grew older, these trips diminished. Dad was a hard worker and Mum went back to school as a teacher. Somehow or other we all carried on, everyone busy with their own lives: Dad promoting his business, Mum supporting him as much as possible, children selfishly trying to enjoy themselves all the time! We *always* sat down at the table together for meals, though. No TV dinners for us. These were the times the family were together to chat and socialise and catch up on our days. I loved that time of family togetherness.

DARK DAYS

In 1970, Mum developed breast cancer. I was 15 years old and on holiday in Romorantin, France, on a school exchange visit with my pen-friend Yannie. I still have the letters I received from Mum throughout the three-week stay. They are full of motherly concern, worrying about me remembering to take my travel sickness pills, describing life at home – but there is no mention of doctors or hospitals, or any other such incidents.

It wasn't until I returned home that I was told Mum had undergone a mastectomy. I knew of cancer at close quarters because my maternal grandma had died from ovarian cancer in our house a couple of years before. Grandma and Grandpa lived with us at that point as Grandpa had had a stroke many years earlier that left him very disabled, paralysed down one side of his body and unable to speak intelligibly. Yet Diane and I were always able to understand exactly what he was saying. Diane would regularly get Grandpa to play snap with her, teaching him how to say 'snap'. To this day, we still have cine film – no sound available though, of Diane pointing patiently and mouthing the words 'say snap'.

Grandma died a long, lingering, destroying death due to the spread of ovarian cancer. The vivid picture that haunted me was of her yellow skin and unseeing, staring eyes; eyes that bulged from a hollow face. I think I was around 12 years old. Grandpa subsequently went into a lovely local home very close to us, and we would visit all the time.

But I knew nothing much about breast cancer. The way I saw it was that Mum's mastectomy had sorted the problem out. You didn't die from a mastectomy, I was certain of that. There was no complaining, just an acceptance of the surgery, and we were shown the prosthetic 'falsie' to insert into her bra to 'even her up'. I had no qualms whatsoever then. Mum was fit and well, and had continued to correspond throughout her hospital stay, brushing off the illness and the surgery as if it didn't exist.

I therefore continued my new-found existence as a lively, fun-loving teenager, giggling my way through life with Linda. Endless silly incidents would have us rolling around with laughter – like the time when we had a competition to see which of us could get the most Tom Thumb drops into their mouth at once. I proudly beat the record, managing to cram a full half pound of the little sweets into my mouth at the bus stop one evening. When the bus arrived, I tried to say 'three please' (the cost of the fare), but the driver could not decipher the unintelligible sounds I was making. I turned to Linda for help, but she was totally useless, crying with laughter. In desperation I opened my mouth very slightly to try to make the request clearer and the pressure of the squashed-in Tom Thumb drops was too much. They started to emit themselves like a machine gun firing bullets. The poor driver, fed up of being in this sticky firing range, told me to 'bugger off down the bus' – an order which I gratefully obeyed, laughing all the way with these wretched things shooting out at all angles. So many stories, such laughs and good times.

Meanwhile the treacherous cancer was invading Mum's body.

The following Easter, Dad arranged a golfing tour of Scotland with a friend of his. Both families went along, although they had better sleeping arrangements than us. Dad had hired a campervan – what an experience! This thing must have been at least 200 years old. We chugged up to Scotland – in the driving rain. Dad played golf at St Andrews – in the driving rain. We set up the sleeping arrangements – in the driving rain. The roof of the campervan lifted up. Two single pull-out beds then appeared in the roof. Diane managed to grab the one on the metal side; I was left with the canvas side. In the driving rain we went to bed.

Canvas leaks!

My sleeping bag was soaked. It was awful. Even my incorrigible sense of humour deserted me. The next night I slept on the floor, curled up round the hideous Elsan toilet. Fortunately, the following day, the hateful vehicle broke down. Hurray! We had to hire a car and join our friends in their B&B. How sensible and what a relief, until we discovered where we were going to stay next.

Our friends' daughter, Penny, had a book aptly entitled *Interesting Places to Stay in Scotland*. She was gleeful about the next proposed stopover. We pulled up at the thirteenth-century mansion and crunched down the eerie, tree-lined gravel drive to the main door, the wind howling and owls hooting. Dad lifted the enormous knocker and, as it crashed back into place, the whole building seemed to resound. Eventually a little old lady opened the creaking door, just as you might have expected in a Vincent Price movie. She welcomed us into a large open hallway with a sweeping staircase leading from it. A suit of armour complete with axe stood at the bottom. We were shown up to our rooms, which were equally scary. Even Mum and Dad by this time had succumbed to the collywobbles. We decided we would all sleep in the same room as a family. Penny did the same with her parents.

Of course, by morning everything looked entirely different. Cocks were crowing and peacocks were strutting around the magnificent yard. Gone was the eerie bleakness of the previous evening, replaced with sheer old-fashioned grandeur; shabby, but still grand.

I had no idea that this would be the last family holiday ever with Mum. This was April 1971. Sadly, Mum's cancer was by now manifesting itself in other parts of her body. She was recommended for radiotherapy in May, from which Dad told us she would get much worse before getting better. And worse she became, getting thinner all the time, and more frail than I had ever seen her. I didn't accompany her on any of these outpatient treatments and I continued living the life of a selfish teenager, petrified of missing any events within our network of friends.

During August, Mum became very ill. I felt really annoyed with the doctors. She ate nothing at all and was losing weight at an alarming rate. Very soon her strong legs were thinner than my young limbs. Why wasn't she in hospital on a drip? How on earth was she ever to get better eating nothing at all? It made no sense to me, because I believed that Dad's proclamation that 'she would become worse before improving' would hold true. Wouldn't it? Didn't grown-ups tell the truth? I realise now that this was Dad's way of protecting us. Also, I doubt Mum had been told she was terminally ill. So, I watched this pitiful decline, interrupted by one short interlude at the local hospital. It was probably a hospice. I, the eternal optimist, believed she was there to build herself up, but to no avail.

Diane and I were kept busy in those last few days while Mum's breathing developed into the hideous death rattle of someone whose cancer has metastasized into the lungs. Dad kept us out of the house most of the time; Mum barely recognised us. The breathing noise was terrifying. That final evening Dad sent us to visit his sister, Aunty Kath, whom both Diane and I adored. She was a droll raconteur, and from an early age, had been one of our favourite babysitters. The evening went along as usual, and it was some relief to be out of the house and away from the constant reminder of my helplessness to relieve Mum's torment in any way.

Aunty Kath rang Dad around nine o'clock, then softly told us that it was time for us to go home. We had no idea at this point that Mum was dead. Dad arranged for us to be collected by someone, I cannot remember who. As we walked into the house, Dad quietly told us he had some very sad news. He held his arms open to cuddle us both, and told us Mum had died. He scarcely got the words out before his own composure collapsed, and the father who had always appeared so strong, now seemed to me to be vulnerable himself. We went into the bedroom before the undertaker came. I saw

Mum lying still, her cheeks pale and sunken, and I suddenly understood the expression, 'they are at peace now'. The insane struggle with life was over for my mummy; no longer did she have to fight the wretched battle to breathe, against the grip of this hateful disease.

I found it hard to believe that she was dead. Of course I realised how poorly she had become, but I still never imagined that this could end in her death. Surely if anyone had suspected death, doctors and hospitals would be working hard to prevent it? I think the shock was too great to absorb in one go. I had optimistically hung on to Dad's earlier announcement that she would get worse before getting better. I believed that totally and never suspected that it would not be true.

Fairly soon, I understood that Dad hadn't wanted us to break down in front of Mum. She had not been told she was dying. Dad told me years later that the consultant had called him in to his office on his own and said, 'I am sorry, but there is nothing more we can do,' and gave Mum just three months to live. How Dad kept a handle on this is amazing. He didn't tell Mum, but kept her going with the same story that she would get worse before improving. This is an unimaginable burden for someone to have to shoulder alone, yet my hero father ran the house, kept his business going, tried to feed the family, and tempt Mum to eat – all the time knowing the dreadful truth. He was so stoical throughout this truly awful period, but I do remember one day seeing him in the kitchen after yet another miserable failed attempt at getting Mum to eat, crying as he threw the food in the bin. Of course, I should have realised the truth, but cancer was just not spoken about in those days so I had such scant knowledge of its terminal nature. Poor Daddy. I so loved and worshipped him and believed in his ability to mend everything for us.

True to the consultant's predictions, Mum died exactly three months after she finished the gruelling radiotherapy. It was 19 August, the day before my parents' wedding anniversary.

Dad set up a bed for all of us in the living room that evening. I was overwhelmed by the constant need to keep going to the toilet. Nerves had really set in. Diane was similarly affected. Aunty Kath stayed too. We were all trying our best to make sense of things, and felt desperate that we couldn't.

The funeral was an almost unreal experience, that left me feeling as if I was just an observer. I don't remember being as upset as I thought I should be, simply because the whole procedure seemed surreal, as if I was just looking on at something that didn't concern me. Mourning and regrets were such a long way away for me. It wasn't until we went into the crematorium's remembrance area after the service and read the messages on the flowers that any of this penetrated at all. I'm sure that if I'd had to watch a coffin being lowered into the ground, that would have jolted my anaesthetised consciousness.

After the funeral, Dad took us to stay with Mum's sister, my Aunty Betty, and her two daughters. They lived in London, so there was plenty to keep us all occupied. We visited the Ideal Home Exhibition and generally, although half-heartedly, played the tourist. I received my O level results in a phone call from a friend. I had passed eight O levels, but there wasn't much jubilation about it. I think numb and disbelieving would be the best way to describe how I felt about it all.

Diane was much younger than I, being just 12 years

old when Mum died. She was always very shy and lacked confidence. None of us spoke much about Mum's illness at the time. What could you say? The sight was pitiful and horrendous but I, always the optimist, looked on each mouthful of food taken as being a good sign. Diane told me many years later that she once found herself thinking, 'What will happen if Mum dies?', then felt guilty for having such thoughts. That is dreadful really, that a 12-year-old should feel guilty for worrying that their mother might die. But that is Diane. Always sweet and pretty, and very shy until she gets to know you.

She told me that she remembers going back to school in September and just feeling lost. I too can remember that feeling, but at 16 years old I also had a social life well and truly in place in addition to family life. It was so much harder for Diane. A neighbour, Mrs Thompson, who lived at the bottom of our garden, had been good to us all throughout this time. She looked after my sister after school until I got off the bus, then we would walk home together. Before she died, Mum had been knitting Diane a green cardigan. Mrs Thompson taught Diane to knit and, between them, they finished this off. It was so precious to Diane, and I think she still has it.

I do regret that we didn't talk about this more at the time. We just didn't dwell on it at all. Dad was amazing. He kept everyone busy, yet it must have been so hard for him. He was in the early days of his own business, with its many financial ups and downs. I always had at least three part-time jobs just so that I could keep up with my own fashion 'must-haves'! Having passed my O levels, I was now starting my A level courses, so I suppose I kept myself pretty much occupied. But, of course, I loved my little sister, and we continued as we always had done, sharing the day-to-day living, which led to much co-operation.

There is one interesting story, so strange that I am unlikely ever to forget it. After Mum died, Dad went the following morning to the home where our grandad, Mum's father, lived. Although Grandpa couldn't speak properly, we knew with great certainty that he could comprehend. He still read the papers, watched TV, and suchlike.

When my father arrived at the small private home, the matron said, even before he had a chance to explain, that Mr Gould (Grandpa) had tried to get out of bed the night before. The regime in the home was that at seven p.m. every evening the staff would undress him and put him to bed with his television on at the foot of the bed. He would stay in bed until seven the following morning. The matron told Dad that the previous night they had heard noises in Grandpa's room. The staff went in at nine o'clock and found him attempting to get up and dress himself.

This was *exactly* the time his daughter – my mother – died. Whatever you believe or not, you do have to agree it was the most amazing coincidence. I still to this day have no idea what to make of it. Neither does Dad.

Shortly after Mum died, I visited our GP with a specific purpose.

'Could breast cancer be hereditary?' I asked. Mum and Grandma had both developed and suffered from it. Grandma had survived breast cancer twice in her forties, but died aged 67 from ovarian cancer.

The GP dismissed my concerns. He said that lightning was unlikely to strike in the same place twice, and was sure it would not happen a third time. I enjoyed his reassurance, but was unable to totally rid myself of the niggling doubts. It was to become a question I would ask my GP at every visit about any other matter. Each time I received the same dismissive answer, and was convinced that he entered 'hypochondriac' in my notes. I didn't, however, let the worry take over my life. If there was to be a problem, it would be far into the future, I thought, but the possibility remained a nagging worry in my mind.

Meanwhile, things continued, as they are wont to do, and we – dad, Diane and I – all tried to rebuild our lives. We muddled through the household chores, and had a cleaning lady once a week. Dad did the shopping and much of the cooking, but we all chipped in. Of course, Mum had not been able to help anyway, for so many weeks prior to her death. All the chores just sort of happened. Ironing, for example, was something we would each do for ourselves as needed. There were no plans or arrangements, we just got on with things as they occurred. The large garden was now bereft of its showjumping course, and as a family we three would spend Sunday mornings in our wellingtons, working away together and trying to keep on top of the gardening.

I remember one of these Sundays in particular. We came inside, ate our roast lunch, which Dad had cooked with our help, and sat and watched that wonderful vintage film, *Random Harvest*. The three of us, still wearing our wellies, were silently sobbing over the soapy, sentimental climax as the kitchen remained in disarray, the pots and dishes unwashed. Around four o'clock there was a knock at the door. Dad, bless him, had invited some family friends for tea and had forgotten all about it. They turned up to an unkempt house, no fire, and a welcome committee sitting in the darkness. No tea, just a kitchen full of pots.

We soon turned it all around though. It's amazing how tolerant and understanding true friends can be. A fire was lit, pots were washed, and the fridge and pantry raided to cobble together something resembling tea. Life began to return to normality.

A few months after Mum died, Dad bought a small travel agency. He had done some printing for the owner, who had lost everything by drinking his profits away, and wheedled Dad into buying the company using the monies he was owed for his printing, in part payment. Dad reluctantly agreed, and there he met Olive, who worked at the counter of this little travel agency.

This meeting turned out to have the most profound significance for all our lives. Olive and Dad started dating, and I remember Dad showing me a shirt she had bought for him at Christmas.

I jokingly said, 'Oh, does she fancy you?', a typically outspoken teenage remark. Dad grimaced at my forthright question, but laughingly conceded that this was possibly so. I was delighted.

They married the following year. Dad was getting his life back. Olive became a wonderful friend to Diane and me. She never had any children, so there were no complications to overcome. We just welcomed this kind, delightful lady into our home, making Dad happy again and bringing order back into our lives. We all got on so well. Olive is one of life's treasures, a wonderful person whom everyone likes. She always told us, 'I'm not going to try to mother you', and we quickly learned to love this lovely lady who brought so much light and happiness back into our home. Dad had looked so poorly himself throughout this time, his own health suffering somewhat while he battled to keep everything going. Not that he was ill, but he looked tired and jaded, which was just not what our dad was about. He was a strong, dependable character who could, in our eyes, cope with everything. I was so happy for him.

Dad and Olive's wedding was hilarious. We had a marquee on the lawn, exactly where my jumps used to stand. The day was very hot and sunny, and everyone seemed to drink far too many toasts. When Olive and Dad left to start their honeymoon, I was unsure if it was my responsibility to call taxis for all the guests who were far too 'happy' to be sitting behind a wheel. I even found our bank manager having a little snooze under the hedge. Some party!

Olive encouraged my singing, for which I am eternally grateful. Much solace can be found through music, and much fun too. Olive introduced me to the world of musical theatre, and I loved every minute of it. She would play our organ at home, which had been Mum's pride and joy. She had a perfect knack for encouraging confidence in myself that I was sadly lacking.

'You have a beautiful voice,' she used to say, and suggested I take up singing lessons.

My very first appearance in a show was in the front row of the chorus of *Mame* when I was about 18. The production and dance routines were fantastic fun, except for the props. We each had a parasol, which formed part of the dance to the title song. This was a massive production number, culminating in the parasols all being opened with precision timing on the very last chorus word, 'Mame'. Throughout the rehearsals, my practice umbrella had caused problems, from refusing to budge to turning itself inside out.

I was unprepared, though, for the pièce de résistance during the actual show week. I thought I had really got the hang of the swift, snappy movement, in time with the others; a grand sweeping gesture – parasol in left hand, action from the right. The first two performances went like clockwork then, on the third evening, I put up the parasol with such a flourish that, instead of just opening, it carried on and flew right off the end of the stick, opened itself out and parachuted back down into the orchestra, leaving me centre stage holding the stick. I was aghast. The audience, meanwhile, thought it was a hoot.

Holidays with Linda resumed. The one that really altered my life was the trip to Benidorm at the age of 16. Oh my goodness! Spanish waiters understood women, and knew just how to pay a compliment; the whole atmosphere everywhere oozed romance, flamenco and excitement. Benidorm old town was just the most romantic place at night, with its small guitar bars and cobbled streets. The view across either bay with the reflected lights from the hotels gleaming in the sea was spectacular. I fell totally under the Spanish romantic spell.

That trip to Benidorm entirely shaped my future. Gone were any ideas of university. What I now wanted to do was become a travel rep and work abroad. I ditched one of my A level courses and swiftly took on two extra O level courses: Spanish and Italian. They were not that easy to learn at the same time due to their similarities, but I passed my Spanish O level in six months. I then used my extended six-week holiday to work in Mallorca as a travel rep. I was 17 years old! In fact, my dad helped fix this up. By now, his little travel agency was running a short season of package holidays to Mallorca, and Dad gave me the opportunity to work during the busy high season. I hastily passed my driving test – a car was necessary for this summer post – and so, off to Mallorca. Sometimes you just have to make things happen!

I arrived at Palma airport and was taken to the tour operator's offices in the heart of the city. I couldn't believe the traffic! I was taken to the rear of the offices and given a map of Santa Ponca, some 20 miles or so away along the coast. I was also handed the car keys. It was rather a disappointing elderly vehicle – an old battered SEAT. In broken English, the operator told me this car had no synchromesh in the gears and I would have to double declutch. What? In the middle of Palma? Four days after passing my driving test? But I gamely jumped in and set off, having no idea how I was going to escape this bustling crazy city in a car that didn't behave with any normality. Four days after passing my driving test I banged, crashed and crunched my way through the gears, and somehow managed to get to the Hotel Pisces in Santa Ponca, which was to be my base for the eight-week stay.

It didn't take a 17-year-old girl very long to suss out the Spanish waiters and be disappointed in the shorter Mallorquin stature. Very few were taller than me, and not one matched up to the delicious Laurence Olivier lookalike I had fallen for in Benidorm. Not to worry; it was hot, beautiful, and I had survived the flight and the haphazard journey. I met my co-worker, Peter Sanders, and found we were to share two vehicles – the other being a motorbike. Hilarious! I had never ridden one in my life, but there is a first time for everything, I guess.

We were to manage five hotels between us. Only a few days after my arrival, Peter asked me to visit the guests at Portals Nous, Hotel Aquamarine. He explained the directions clearly. I must head back towards Palma for around 10 miles, and then turn sharp right down to Portals Nous. 'Fine,' I said. 'Turning right should be easy, given I am already driving on the right-hand side of the road.' Driving? Peter shook his head. 'Sorry,' he said, 'you need to take the motorbike.' Evidently Peter had a hot date with a particularly pretty blonde girl who had just arrived, and he was anxious to drive her out to some romantic destination along the coast. Hmmm, I thought. Well, OK. I'll manage. It must just be like riding a bike, but a bit faster. Easy. Piece of cake!

I set off, wearing no bike gear whatsoever but just a thin T-shirt, shorts, and long (blonde at that time) hair blowing in the breeze. Passing lorries tooting and waving, me thoroughly enjoying the whole experience. I saw the sign for Portals Nous, with a hairpin bend indicated. Peter had said it was 'sharp right', but I was unprepared for the actual turn. I halted, and then slowly released the brake, as not only was it sharp right, but downhill too! The bike took on a mind of its own. It refused to go slowly and, completely out of control, sped across the road, hitting the stone wall and leaping over like a crazed motocross expert, careering through a ditch, and finally lodging itself in the chicken wire separating a little farmyard from the roadside. I hurtled for some of the time as though one with the bike, but eventually the momentum was too great and we parted company like a cartoon scene: the bike falling to earth and crashing onto its side, while I completed a human cannonball stunt, only thwarted from reaching record-breaking distances by the mesh wire fence.

I slowly picked myself up, wondering which was most damaged, me or the silly bike. How dare it take off on its own! I managed to make it down to the Hotel – on foot. I was in marginally better shape than my mode of transport.

The guests were patiently waiting in reception for me, their courier. I was there to book their trips; deal with erratic plumbing in their bathrooms, and generally pander to every whim. I put my sunglasses on to hide the bash on my eye (I eventually discovered a small chip in my cheekbone), and sorted things out for them. The next step was to get back to Santa Ponca, somehow or other. I called our hotel, and luckily Peter was in reception. His 'hot date' had not quite worked out as anticipated, so my news just about finished his day off for him. He drove over to pick me up, surveying the wreckage that had been our motorbike, and only then expressed concern for me. I have no idea where that bike went, and didn't care either . . . for all I know, it might still be there!

Working in Mallorca at 17 years old was marvellous fun. Booking trips to barbecues and nightclubs was our responsibility, and the guests loved them. I pretty soon realised the best way of ensuring a trouble- and moan-free week was to make a darn good job of the champagne reception on the first day. It was of utmost importance to get everyone totally plastered if possible; then they would relax and have a good time whatever happened. I usually bore the brunt of the jollities, managing to get myself thrown in the pool most evenings. They were good times.

I went back to school and finished my A levels, then

returned for a further season in Mallorca at Cala d'or. Once again it was a charming place, but the first weekend was a total nightmare as the newly built hotel was not quite ready. After the initial panics, the holidays went ahead smoothly. I worked in two hotels on my own, which was a real responsibility, but somehow I muddled through.

This phase was followed by a return to home again, and lots of different jobs followed. I was by now determined to buy a horse and a car. Vehicles have since been the bane of my life. I bought my first horse, and eventually bought a small pony and started to give riding lessons myself. I needed a job that would leave me the daytimes free to 'school' and look after my horses, so I utilised my school qualifications to their full capacity by applying for, and getting a job with, the the local co-operative dairy.

I became a milkman!

This job suited me perfectly. We could start at three-thirty a.m. and were paid for eight hours' work, but it was up to the individual if they rushed round and finished quickly. Learning the rounds and how to manage the crates was about the most challenging element. The first hot day on my own I decided that perhaps this wouldn't be quite as easy as I thought. With three streets left to complete, and having really lost the pattern from the 'round book', I found myself with all the remaining full milk crates in the centre of the milk float, all the empties piled up round the outsides, preventing me reaching the milk.

I had several disasters during my career as a milkman. I was forever reversing into posts, and, once, I went round a corner and lost the entire three crates of 'school milk'; those little third-of-a-pint bottles – 63 of them. That really was difficult to fix, as the dairy understandably only had a limited number of these bottles. I had to appease the irate teacher by offering to go to a local shop and buy paper cups.

The worst disaster of all was the time I forgot to unplug my electric cart from the battery charger it had been attached to all night. The dairy had a low concrete wall on which stood the rows of giant battery chargers. After the round was finished, these milk carts would be plugged in to recharge their enormous batteries.

Having loaded my cart with its 43 crates of milk in record time, I jumped in and reversed away from the wall, totally forgetting to unplug it from its charger. The cart jumped into action, pulling the battery charger off the wall with it and crashing to the ground.

'They cost £3,000,' wailed the supervisor.

Oh dear. I was abject with apologies while the rest of the milkmen – men, of course – were helpless with laughter. After destroying nine posts, two cars, umpteen crates of milk and a battery charger, I was expecting to get the sack, but it never happened.

Pretty soon, the local riding school, Maywood Farm in Risley, employed me as a live-in teacher. The kids and I got on famously, as I was always up for joining in with all their antics. The riding school also doubled as a livery stables; many kids had their ponies stabled there and would turn up every day, particularly during school holidays, to look after them and generally mess about on the farm all day. In reality, I guess for those parents we also made rather useful crèche facilities, as there was always a responsible adult around to oversee everything.

Here I met Jeremy Measures, through his daughter Corrine who had a pony stabled at Maywood. Jeremy and his wife had split up and Corrine had stayed with her father. He would drop her off at the farm before going to work. Corrine and I became very close and she was certainly instrumental in my eventually marrying her father. He was much older than me but we naturally became a family, Corrine adopting me as a replacement mother. We would go to horse shows together. Corrine was a very talented rider and I soon became involved in furthering her abilities and finding many suitable ponies for her to compete on.

Jeremy and I had a similar sense of humour, but chiefly it was our comfort in family matters that drew us together. 'Companionable' I think describes it. Dad and Olive by this time were living in Mallorca, Diane was married, and I found something homely about this ready-made family.

We had a small wedding since money, as usual, was tight – most of it by this time being spent on ponies! Horseriding really is not an inexpensive hobby in either time or money, but it was our lives. From first thing in the morning, going to the livery yard, mucking out the ponies, feeding them and exercising them, each day was mapped out. Anyone involved with horses will tell you it becomes an obsession. It has to, to warrant the amount of time and money the hobby costs. Of course, this is how we had married. I moved into Jeremy's house in Long Eaton and within a year gave birth to our gorgeous daughter, Becky.

All through my pregnancy, I was convinced it was a girl. So was Jeremy. I was really excited at actually having a baby of my own, as I had become a surrogate mum to so many of the kids at the riding school. I loved children, and knew how to entertain them. I knew about fun and excitement, picnics and adventures; and children warmed to me. I was very concerned that something might go wrong during the pregnancy, but I managed to keep riding and working until I was in my seventh month. At this time I was teaching at Elvaston Castle Riding Stables. One weekend I was taking a hack (ride) out round the park. The horse I was on was spooked by something, and set off with its head between its knees, bucking like crazy. Somehow or other I managed to stay on and get it back under control, but it frightened me immensely. I decided enough was enough. Just looking after Corrine's ponies was more than sufficient in my last few weeks of pregnancy.

I resist the urge to tell you the gory details of a three-day labour to produce this beautiful wide-eyed little girl. I found the whole experience incredible, and was amazed that I was capable of growing and producing something so perfect! Three days of labour was such a long time. The horseriding throughout the pregnancy had made my muscles strong and reluctant to give way, and I was truly exhausted. But just watching this little bundle in the cot at the side of my bed while the surgeon sewed me back up was remarkable. I knew immediately what to call her: Rebecca Helen, Helen being my mum's middle name. She didn't sleep, but stared wide-eyed, hardly blinking. She reminded me of the birthday cards that were around at the time. Huge eyes set very wide apart, and a tiny nose and mouth. Seven pounds, eight ounces of perfection – and of course I am totally unbiased!

Becky looked so innocent, yet she was quick to work

out just who was boss in that household, immediately having the attention of three adoring people and never being short of a pick-up or a cuddle. Oh yes, from about six days old Becky knew exactly how to manage these people. I was totally besotted with her and adored her. I could not bear to hear her cry, and found myself completely unable to be firm over this. If Becky cried to be picked up, then I was happy to do just that. It was weeks before I trusted anyone else to babysit, even for an hour or so. A neighbour had recently lost her lovely baby girl through the inexplicable 'cot death' syndrome, which made me neurotic lest the same should happen.

We were inseparable, Becky and I, and remain so to a certain extent even now. I think I had a completely different relationship with Becky than my own mother and I had. Mum wasn't really the cuddly type, although she showed her love in the care and attention she bestowed upon us, whereas I am open about my feelings. I love to hug people and to be hugged myself. Becky has inherited this from me and we are similar in many ways.

Corrine was an excellent rider. We would all take off for anywhere that a weekend's showjumping could be found. Becky, Corrine, the two girls who helped with the ponies, and I would pile into the horsebox, an elderly Lambourn, with a maximum speed of around 35 miles per hour . . . eventually. We had such fun, sleeping in the cab and cooking sausages on the little Calor gas cooker. It was an amazing childhood for Becky too. She spent much of her time with me, but had a gregarious upbringing, associating with children of all ages. She was spoilt by many of them, loved and hugged endlessly. At the age of two, Becky had her own pony, Marigold, whom we used to take to the shows with us. We all found it so much easier to pop Becky on Marigold and lead her around than push an unwieldy pushchair through inches of mud. Becky adored her pony, and I guess I was just reliving my childhood through her.

Becky very quickly showed a love for animals. We had a cat called Sooty, which unfortunately went missing. A neighbour told us that they had seen a dead cat at the side of the road, around a hundred yards from where we lived. Hating the idea, I had to go, complete with shovel and bin liner, to inspect this corpse and bring it home for a proper burial. I dreaded this. I pulled up at the side of the road, and saw the dead cat. I shuddered but nevertheless did as I was bid. I arrived home and we prepared for a proper burial, including a full service – the works!

The next morning, there on the kitchen windowsill, was Sooty meowing to be let in! I nearly collapsed. Had he risen from the dead? I quickly let him in, inspecting him for traces of soil, then rushed down the garden. Indeed, the burial place was totally undisturbed.

Everyone was so joyful, until I suddenly thought – if this is Sooty, whose cat is buried in my garden? Whoever owned the dead cat ought to know its whereabouts. I decided I must ring the police station and confess to having stolen a dead cat from the side of the road and buried it in my garden! This was too much for the desk sergeant. He really thought he had a crank on the phone – ringing up and confessing to burying stolen dead cats.

We had various pets, including a dog called Judy, who obsessively followed me everywhere. She never needed a lead, as she was at heel continuously. We had cade lambs in the garden – lambs that had lost their mothers. It almost became a menagerie.

Becky first went to school in Risley, a very select area. It was known as the stockbroker belt of Nottingham. Becky's school had no more than 65 pupils in the entire school, infants and juniors, at any one time. We lived a couple of miles away. By this time, my life had progressed to trying to earn enough money from horses to keep us all in competitive riding, while managing a toddler with whom I was totally besotted.

The cost of keeping horses was incredible, in addition to running lorries and attending shows, and it was a hobby for the select few. However, I was not going to be thwarted, so I continued teaching, running a small livery yard, and generally working all day and night on the horses, breaking them in and looking after them. I felt that with Corrine's ability, she deserved every chance I could give her. In 1984 we set a goal to qualify for the Christy Beaufort Junior Showjumper of the Year at the Horse of the Year Show at Wembley. This involved having an appropriately qualified JA pony in order to even compete in these events. They cost a fortune: £10,000 was nothing to pay for a pony of this calibre even in those days. We had to grow our own almost. Through buying and selling I eventually found one that could do the job for us. We qualified for the regional finals of this competition to be held in Scotland, some 265 miles away.

The journey took over nine hours. There was myself, Becky, Corrine and the two girls who helped us, going off on this jaunt. Financially, it was nigh on impossible, but I gamely loaded the lorry with enough sausages to feed an army, and enough petrol to get us there. From then on we needed to sleep in the cab of the lorry. Becky did best out of this. She was small enough to sleep on the front double seat. Corrine and the girls had sleeping bags on the floor behind the seats. I slept in the driver's seat, which at least did recline slightly, with my feet up on the steering wheel. I now question how much I could have enjoyed this amount of discomfort. We were driven by the desire to succeed where only those better off financially could usually manage. I really wanted Corrine to have this opportunity. And yes, the kid inside me still enjoyed the adventure. Three days without a bank statement or bill was most enjoyable and welcome!

It paid off. Corrine and her pony Drumacre Twist (Jake, his pet name) qualified for Wembley! So thrilling, and the culmination of a dream to succeed. We had managed to get to Wembley as competitors. Astounding!

We came away from Wembley with a fourth place rosette. We sold Jake to a very nice family and tried to pay off some of the debts.

Money was nevertheless really tight, while my vehicles had slumped into a real decline. One Mini, practically held together by a thread, had no suspension left at all. One day it hit a bump in the road, which was nothing more than a small road repair, and both its front headlights fell out! I just calmly carried on home, as the lights were still attached by the wires. But the two-mile journey from Becky's school necessitated a reliable vehicle, and my Cortina required the battery to be removed every morning and charged for half an hour before it would even attempt to turn the engine. Its spark plugs needed a pre-heating session in the oven if the weather was remotely wet or misty.

Eventually I was down to using our lorry, an old Ford Transit horsebox, as a car. It had an engine that could have auditioned for a starring role in *Last of the Summer Wine*, as it could backfire with the best. Becky learned to dread arriving at school. Other mums would be chatting calmly at the school gates when we emerged from Risley Lane, announcing our uncouth arrival in the most noisy manner! We were frequently late, but Becky's school mistress always knew to include Becky on the register – after all, she could hear us as we back-fired our way on the last-half mile of the journey. Luckily enough, by this time I was considered to be a respected horsewoman and trainer. Many of the mums booked me as a private tutor for their children's riding lessons, or asked me to help them find a suitable pony.

Jeremy and I parted when Becky was six years old. There was no animosity whatsoever over the split. Our marriage had produced a wonderful daughter and a step-mum for Corrine. We were probably drawn together initially by circumstances rather than a passionate love affair. Corrine had now moved in with her boyfriend and had stopped riding. Becky was now the 'rider' in the family, and I had carried on buying, selling, schooling and breaking in horses and ponies. I even managed to sell a couple of ponies to the famous showjumping Whittaker brothers for their children. Jeremy and I had been living together, but we'd really been leading separate lives, which eventually led to the split. Jeremy met up with an old flame whom he married once we had divorced. Everything was very civilised. Jeremy had Becky on alternate weekends, and was free to contact her whenever he wished.

I met Chris Watson at a horse show (hardly surpris-ing) and we very quickly got together. Chris was brilliant with Becky. He made such a fuss of her, and treated her as his own.

He was a policeman, who ran the mounted section in Nottinghamshire. Chris had separated from his wife. He had two grown-up children, 18-year-old Mark, who was in the army, and Johanne, shortly to go to teacher training college. I knew them both through our mutual 'horsey' friends. Mark, in particular, was a very brave rider, who would tackle anything at all. He helped me with some of the more difficult ponies. Chris was a tremendous practical joker, and life was happy. We had the horses in common, and many mutual friends.

We married when Becky was eight years old. Becky was tremendously excited. Although this was to be a registry office wedding, she nevertheless wanted a pretty bridesmaid dress. And why not? The dress my daughter chose was white and lacy and, of course, she looked adorable – like a bride herself. I plumped for a red, slim-fitting suit – incredibly flattering to the figure – and also wore the tallest stilettos in creation. They looked fabulous, but felt awful after about 10 minutes.

The wedding was great fun. We enjoyed a luncheon with just our immediate families, who included several Michaels and a couple of Marks. My maiden name was Watson, so almost half of the place names at the table were Mr M Watson, which of course caused the hilarity of pairing the right 'Mr M' with the relevant partner. After this wonderful meal, we all trooped back to our house until the evening do at Moor Farm, to which we had invited our many friends from the horse world.

When the time came to move off for the night event, Dad and Olive made a few excuses about staying behind for a while to do the washing up. I understood. I expect they were just glad of an hour of peace and quiet with a pot of tea. We left them with the house keys.

The evening party, what I remember of it, was lovely. The taxi arrived around one in the morning to take us home. It had been a glorious March day, with not a cloud in the sky, but the evening was cold and frosty. The taxi driver set us down, emptying the boot of the dozens of wedding presents onto the front lawn. Chris felt in his pocket then looked at me.

'Keys?' he asked.

I shook my head. I had a tiny clutch bag with certainly no room for a bunch of keys. Realisation dawned on us both at the same time. Dad and Olive, now back home in Leicestershire, 60 miles away, must have them. As usual I got the giggles, but we looked round the house and finally found one very small window whose latch wasn't fastened. Using a mixture of my highly polished, specially-grown fingernails and a one-penny coin, we prised open the window. My wedding diet had been exceptionally effective and hence I managed to climb through the small space. My immaculate red suit, complete with pencil skirt, wasn't your usual house-breaking apparel, but needs must. I remember thinking wryly that most brides are carried over the threshold, not posted head-first in the most undignified manner through a nine-inch window.

Becky had been delightedly planning where we could all go for 'our' honeymoon, and eventually chose Center Parcs in Nottingham. For anyone who hasn't enjoyed one of these action-packed breaks, let me tell you they are great fun. After the initial unloading of suitcases and other gear, all cars are banned to the far-off car parks. Bicycles are available for hire to cycle round the gorgeous trails of Sherwood Forest within the enormous complex. We spent much of our time teaching Becky to ride a bike, and spent hours in the water dome and water rapids that both Becky and I adored. By the end of our five-day stay, though, Becky was battered and bruised from falling off her bike and then fighting the strong currents of the water rapids. I was convinced that people would wonder who or what on earth I had married, to get my child into this state. Chris, however, was marvellous with Becky and, as I said, treated her as his own.

MOVING ON

Our love of the horses and my earlier romance with the charming Derbyshire Peak District had a profound effect on the subsequent chain of events.

One rainy Sunday afternoon, we were having a particularly unsuccessful day at a horse show, so we decided to abandon the event and take a trip to the Peak District. I had an old copy of the *Derbyshire Times* in the car, advertising a barn with three acres for sale in Over Haddon. We decided to take a look, even though we had no prospects of purchasing it, but the dream was fun. The barn was delightful. The field ran down into Lathkildale from its back door. There was no planning permission and it formed Lot Four of several lots of Lathkil Farm.

As I am the eternal optimist, I contacted the agents, Bagshaws, the very next morning. They told me that the guide price was £80–100,000 for the barn with the small field, but that the main farm itself, complete with 220 acres and 450,000 litres of milk quota, was expected to fetch £450–500,000.

There was no way I could even consider buying

something like this, yet I was determined to think up a way of doing just that – not to make any money, but just to find a way to move into the area I loved and have a small amount of land on which to keep our horses. The only way I could see was to sell much of the property before purchasing it. So, I evolved a plan to sell off the milk quota and some of the land to neighbouring farmers.

Over the next few weeks, I focussed on researching which farmers owned which fields and who among them might be interested in purchasing more land at a relatively cheap price. The farmers treated me with caution, understandably. I chose to use local solicitors in Bakewell for the contracts, so that they would feel more at ease. Sadly, despite my good idea, the farm fetched £600,000 at auction, way out of our price range.

Never daunted by a small setback, I decided I had learnt from the experience. The people who had bought Lathkill Farm actually had a farm of their own to sell. Situated in Arbor Low, it was a much smaller affair – 150 acres and a slightly smaller milk quota – but, nevertheless, a similar proposition. And this time I wasn't making it up as I went along.

Arbor Low is a 4,000-year-old stone circle in the heart of the Midlands. Indeed it is the largest henge in the UK, but the stones now lie in a collapsed condition. The farm effectively acted as gatehouse to this prehistoric site, which was an ancient monument protected by English Heritage. This site was of constant interest to tourists, travellers, scholars, worshippers and mystics; it was also a popular venue for pagan festivals.

I visited the owners of this property, explaining

frankly what I was after, and they gave me the details of all the neighbours, which fields joined on to which, and so on. I visited these neighbours and, eventually, struck a mutually amicable deal to sell some land to three of them. It really became a win-win situation for all concerned: the seller, the other purchasers, and me. The local solicitor soon got contracts in place, subject to the overall purchase, so in effect we never bought anything before selling. It worked like a dream this time. We kept 50 acres and continued the tenancy of a further 50 acres adjoining, selling off around 80 acres. The farmer kept the milk quota in negotiations after the auction. The only problem was we had taken on a mortgage of over £100,000 at interest rates of 15.4 per cent. Not funny.

We moved into the farm on 10 October 1990, and our first night there nearly drove me away. The house seemed to be completely overrun with mice. Having such a passion for the white pet variety had hardly prepared me for the scuffling and rapid movements of the rodents that appeared to inhabit every nook and cranny. In the morning, I dispatched Chris to the local farm suppliers in Bakewell with strict instructions to spend every last penny on Neosorexa or other such vermin eliminators. When he came back, we put little piles of these blue pellets literally everywhere. As the days wore on, the consumption of these piles of 'mouse-food' appeared to be in recession. Then the smell arrived: cabbages. The smell of dead mice is just so similar to the smell of rotten cabbages one might almost wonder if they were of the same family. Chris spent much of the first few days on rodent detection and elimination. Despite these rather unpleasant challenges, nothing detracted from the excitement and fulfilment of how we came to be in our new home.

I set to, working the farm. Since we had few funds to buy much in the way of equipment and stock, we took on 'wintering' of other people's cattle in the enormous sheds. As everyone knows, I never do anything by halves so, pretty soon, what with our own calves as well, I was looking after 350 cattle each day, feeding them and cleaning out. The japes I had over these experiences could cover an entire book in themselves. I'm afraid my knowledge of caring for horses, teaching riding, breaking in and schooling ponies, in no way prepared me for the husbandry of 350 cattle!

The first winter saw fantastic snowfalls. In early December, the blizzards were immense and relentless. We woke up to find the 200-square-foot cowshed completely covered by a snowdrift. The snow was up to our first-floor bathroom window, which became the only way out of the house. We managed to squeeze out of the small frame to stand on top of a 15-foot drift. The whole experience was totally surreal. We created steps down the snowdrift into the back door; the next task was attending to all the animals.

The horses were still 'living out' at this time, complete with rugs, in our largest field. I have never known anything like our efforts to find them. Since then, I know what a 'whiteout' is. Chris and I could neither see nor hear each other due to the sheer intensity of the blizzard. We very quickly turned back to get properly prepared. Although we were in our own field, it was terrifying. We fastened scarves over our faces to help us breathe and then roped ourselves together so that we didn't lose each other. After a fruitless attempt we gave up. There was absolutely no chance of finding anything out there. All we could do was leave the field gate open and the door ajar into the big cattle shed in the hope that if the horses decided to return, they would find the food and shelter for themselves. At the far end of the field was a small wooded area which we assumed they must have found, and we knew they were well rugged up, but this didn't stop the worry.

The next task was to find a way to get food and water through the snow for around 300 beasts. We climbed up and down our man-made steps into the house, carrying buckets of water for the hungry and thirsty animals. We also had several calves in the stables around the house yard, all of whom needed warm milk mixed from large bags of powder. The calves were constantly anxious, and made even more so because we had to lower ourselves into the stables through the top doors. That was after a fight too; shovels were no match for this quantity of snow. What a battle . . .

At the end of a long and wearying day we collapsed indoors, spent from our day's activities, but experiencing a warm sense of satisfaction at having battled successfully against the elements. Every one of the animals was warm, fed and watered. Thankfully, by evening, the horses had eventually heard our calls, and thundered down the field into the cowshed where they were happily munching on the bales of hay in there. Horses and cattle coexist comfortably as if they know that in such times one just has to get on with the other. The only problem unsolved was the whereabouts of the small flock of sheep we had assembled since our arrival just six weeks earlier. Where they were was anyone's guess, but the neighbouring farmers reassured us that they would be fine.

The next morning it was a different world; magical and sparkling blue. Not a cloud in the blue sky which was reflected in the snow. Utterly beautiful. The day's tasks still seemed fairly daunting. We could now see the enormity of the drifts and the extreme problems attached to feeding several hundred hungry animals; but the beauty of the scenery made it worthwhile.

After the initial battles with frozen water pipes, we decided to 'play hunt the sheep'. We were almost at the stage of giving up when I noticed a couple of black pointed objects, sticking up from a drift in the far corner of their field. We shot over there as fast as is possible in knee-deep snow, curious to see what this was. I was amazed to find it was a pair of ears! Sheep's ears! We dug furiously to find they belonged to the top sheep in a pyramid of sheep, acting as an air vent. The entire motley flock of 32 variegated sheep had been buried under the snow. All prepared to be buried alive, with the responsibility of the one on the top tier to keep its head up, creating a channel for air to reach them all for as long as possible.

As we pulled them out one by one, we noticed how warm they had kept themselves, huddled together in their igloo. They merely shook themselves and wandered off as if this was an everyday occurrence. Incredibly, none of them was the worse for wear and all produced baby lambs the following spring.

That day was perhaps one of the most magical days of my life. Later that morning, Bernard, our nearest neighbour from half-a-mile away, appeared, walking across one of our fields. He had a small sack of potatoes slung over his back, and carried a milk churn in his hand. As we let him in, via our super-efficient snow steps, he set down these provisions, then reached into the pocket of his dark donkey jacket and fetched out a small bottle of whisky. We sat drinking steaming mugs of tea round our large kitchen table, listening to Bernard regaling us with 'snow' tales from his lifetime of living in the Derbyshire Peak District. That day I learned something about true neighbourliness.

Life at Arbor Low and its renowned stone circle was palpably different from anything I had ever known. The pace of life was so much slower, yet there was lots of work to be done caring for the animals. The hippies would trek through the farmyard each Midsummer's Eve to welcome in the Solstice. Everyone had their own beliefs, but it was always peaceful. The very first year, we were visited by a gentleman who claimed he had been sent by 'Arthur' to find his sword and then turn on the earth's energies again. In his day job, he was the front-desk clerk at a local police station! He said that, many years before, the earth was being pillaged so the 'powers that be' turned down the earth's energies. He had received a 'calling' to perform the reversal ritual, and wished to do this at daybreak on 21 June, the Summer Solstice. I had no objections to whatever he was planning, provided it was sedate, which he assured me it would be.

That Solstice they all arrived, along with several hundred others – some on their own, and others in groups. One or two had drums, the bongo type, which they planned to thump all night, welcoming in the dawn. The leader arrived with his posse of ladies, all resplendent in white, hooded cloaks. They made their way up to the stone circle.

Approaching dawn, curiosity got the better of me. 'The earth's energies' team sprang into action around five minutes before daybreak. They positioned themselves in four outer points of the circle, with their leader in the centre holding the magnificent sword aloft, pointing towards the heavens. He looked up and started to chant 'Arthur, Arthur, Arthur' until eventually several joined in with him. His ladies dramatically walked towards the centre stone in carefully choreographed moves as he lowered the sword and put it into the soil. He attempted to rotate it a quarter turn, but the dry soil was unyielding, so he satisfied himself with 'cutting the turf' through 90 degrees.

The following weekend, early on the Saturday morning, we had the mother and father of thunderstorms. Our farmhouse was so high, almost on the apex of a hill, that the lightning was terrifyingly close. We not only unplugged the television and various other appliances, but switched the electricity off altogether. One immense lightning flash and its accompanying thunderclap scared us silly. Blue flashes leapt across the internal walls, and although the electricity was off, the kitchen lights flashed on momentarily. Well, that was it! Out we all piled into the car and made for the bottom of the drive, hoping to find safety in the rubber tyres and reduction in altitude. Eventually the storm passed.

We returned to the house to find all the telephones dead. Chris examined one of them and found the insides had completely melted! We called BT engineers, who came out a couple of days later and gave a logical explanation as to why the kitchen lights had flashed on. Evidently, a telephone has a capacitor which stores electricity and enables the ring-tone. Clearly, the lightning had struck the house, or at least the phone lines, and got into this capacitor thing, circulating around the many extensions, and shorting across to the electricity wires, hence the blue flashes and the kitchen lights playing at haunted houses.

Later that day, a policeman called to see if everything had been peaceful the previous weekend at the Solstice. I teasingly replied that it had, but Mr Earth's Energies, his front-desk man, had something to answer for. Turning the energies up like that had scared me to death and he could jolly well return here straight away and turn them back down again!

With that, the policeman left, and within less than an hour, Mr Earth's Energies turned up. Well, he didn't just turn up, he screeched up our long drive in a cloud of dust. He was charged with excitement at hearing this news and wanted to know exactly what had happened. It made his day, since he was convinced that this was all his doing, and nothing at all to do with high pressures, weather systems, or the fact that Arbor Low was elevated and could easily attract lightning. To him, he had achieved his purpose. The earth's energies were now well and truly restored.

Farming continued to throw up one hysterical disaster after another. Our neighbours were mildly amused at the antics of what they saw as hapless townsfolk, trying hard but constantly getting themselves into a tangle. One day, a tourist on his way up to visit the stone circle, knocked on the door. He asked me if I knew that there was a sheep in the slurry pit. The slurry pit is effectively a tank of cow poo; it's generally kept runny by using a giant stirrer on the back of a tractor to whisk it occasionally in order to stop a crust forming. And it was in this very tank and its contents that one of our stupid sheep was practicing to become the next Mark Spitz.

What to do?

I knew I couldn't leave the idiotic thing swimming round in that all day, so I had to get out the loader tractor, with its front-loader arms and the pronged fork on the ends, then drive down the sloped side into the tank, which currently had about three feet of this inglorious mixture in it. Stage one worked fine. I made it. The next hazardous action was to try and scoop up the sheep onto the fork, lift it up, and drive it to the edge, all without hurting it.

I manoeuvred the tractor close to the animal. The slurry was too high for me to open the tractor door, so with great dread I climbed out of the window and crawled along the loader arms, mindful of the turgid fate waiting for me below if I fell off. I reached into the slurry for the silly sheep and pulled it onto the tractor fork, settling it on there as best I could. Surprisingly, it did co-operate up to that point. The next task was for me to crawl, in reverse, back up the steel arms and negotiate the difficulty of climbing through the window.

By now, I had a crowd of spectators who – until that moment – had thought the most entertaining part of their day would be a visit to the old stone circle. I tentatively lowered the hydraulic tractor arm and let the sheep off once more onto terra firma. I was filled with elation as I reversed back out of this mess, and just managed to get both myself and the tractor back out of the tank when, guess what?

You got it.

The stupid sheep jumped back in again!

This time, different tactics were used, and I managed to reach it from the side, with the able assistance of the only useful member of the growing crowd, who were by now helpless with laughter.

Becky thinks she had an idyllic childhood. Our farming neighbours were wonderful, and the whole area had a real community spirit. The school, Monyash Primary School, with a grand total of 30 children, was even smaller than the school Becky had moved from. She was picked up from the end of our long farm drive every morning. I made lots of friends among the other mums, who delighted in making us welcome.

The following summer we took the children on long walks, complete with rucksacks full of sandwiches, to explore the gorgeous Derbyshire Peaks and Dales. I rediscovered my love for the exciting Enid Blyton-style adventures, even though I was now in my mid-thirties. I loved getting Becky and her friends up really early in the winter, well before it was light, and taking them out. I would carry a huge rucksack containing primus stoves and pans clattering away, and bulging with bread rolls and sausages for frying. We would drive up to Stanton Moor or the Roaches and I would make the children walk along the rugged footpaths until we found a really great place to pitch camp. They would play hide and seek or explore the surroundings while I got on with making great big mugs of hot steaming tea and frying sausage sandwiches on a primus. There really is very little to beat the smell of food cooked in the open, especially when you have walked far enough to become exceedingly ravenous. Becky still reminisces about those walks with her old school friends.

One evening, around eleven o'clock, I heard cars pull into the car park at the bottom of the drive. I watched as more than 20 people, all carrying candles, trooped up the pathway through the snow, past the farmhouse and went through the fields to Arbor Low. Slightly nervous, and having already had the police assure me I could ring anytime, I did just that. Not because it was an emergency, but merely to reassure myself because as I was on my own that night.

In due course, one of the Bakewell patrol policemen turned up. He said the cars all looked very nice, mostly recent models, but he would go up to the stone circle to see what was going on. I told him about the candle procession, to which in his gloriously broad Derbyshire accent, he replied, 'Eeh, it'll be one of them there rituals.'

I accompanied him through the light layer of snow, a mere four to six inches high, to the stone circle, and my helpful policeman noticed a large patch of red in the snow. Of course, thinking sacrifices and suchlike, he demanded of the 20 or so people who were at that point sitting happily on the centre stones, 'Now then – what you lot up to?' They were all very warmly but smartly dressed and one lady asked what he meant.

He pointed to the offending red stain in the snow and asked, 'What's all this then?'

The lady responded immediately, 'Oh, it's just Sainsbury's red wine,' and produced the bottle. They all then realised what it had looked like and were quick to explain what everything was about. It was the Pagan Festival of Imbolc.

'In many areas of the Celtic world,' explained the lady, 'this was the fire feast of Brighid, the Irish goddess of hearth and home. She is the keeper of the flame, the protector of the home, and a goddess of holy wells and springs. At Imbolc, we acknowledge her many aspects, especially that of her role as a deity of transformation.

As the world awakes from the dark slumber of winter, it is time to cast off the chill of the past and welcome the warmth of spring.'

The ritual involved setting up an altar with symbols, which included a Brigid's cross, some potted daffodils or crocuses, red and white ribbon, fresh twigs, and lots of candles. Then everyone should share a cup of milk and some oats or oatcake. Looking this up, I didn't find any reference to Sainsbury's red wine. That, presumably, was a 'little extra'.

REVELATIONS

Life at Arbor Low had taken on a totally different aspect from what I had expected. The reason to move to a farm was to have some land to further concentrate on the horses, but it just didn't work out like that. We slowly got out of the 'horsey' loop and became immersed in farming.

The local village pub in Monyash was a general meeting place for adults and kids. The tiny village had little else; the nearest shop was five miles away. Hence, The Bull's Head at Monyash became very much the community hub. It was in this very place that I coincidentally met up with my mum's family again. One evening, a gentleman looked across at me and said, 'It's Wendy, isn't it?' I knew I recognised him, but only vaguely. His name was David and he had married my mother's cousin's daughter.

What David then told me was to have the most profound effect on my life. His wife, Jennifer, he said, had suffered breast cancer twice, in both breasts. The first was when she was 32, and the second time, six years later. Jen's sister had died of breast cancer at 38, and her 67-year-old mother had recently developed the disease, as had a cousin aged 48. Jen's aunty had contracted breast cancer when she was 40, but had survived and was then almost 80.

To be honest, I was aghast. I had repeatedly visited the GP over the past 20 years, always asking the same critical question: 'Could breast cancer be hereditary?' And always receiving the same casual answer ('Of course not') from whichever GP was trying to appease me. Now I found that not only were Mum and Grandma affected, but seemingly all our female relatives.

We hastily arranged a meeting with Jennifer. I brought along pens, paper, and an iron determination to ascertain the exact link. Jen hadn't changed at all really, during the 20 or so years since I had last seen her. Our detective work seemed really very authentic, thanks to the ironic coincidence that, while my name was Watson, Jennifer's was Holmes. Jennifer really did not know that my mother and grandmother had both had breast cancer. In fact, my gran had it in both breasts, although she died 20 years later from ovarian cancer. Putting it all together, our findings were conclusive. It was blindingly obvious to anyone that, in our family, breast cancer was indeed hereditary.

With these latest findings I shot off to my new GP, Malcolm Bradbury, at Hartington. I gave him my family tree and implored him, 'Please don't tell me like my previous GPs that this is not hereditary as I would have to say I don't believe you.' He took no more than a nanosecond to examine the evidence and return my gaze. Quietly, he agreed. This was indeed an appalling family history. By this time I was just pleased he agreed with me.

I said to him, 'Okay, what can I do to *prevent* myself from developing the disease?'

He replied that there was nothing I could do, but it was of utmost importance to catch it as early as possible. That would give the best chance of survival. He said he would write and arrange a mammogram for me, but at the age of 37 this was not considered reliable due to the high density of young breast tissue. The mammograms could not be viewed as conclusive; they might miss a small breast cancer and offer false reassurance whereas, in fact, a breast cancer was just not visible due to the breast density.

Meanwhile I was relieved to be taken seriously. Dr Bradbury told me to check myself regularly, a task which was totally impossible for me. I had such a phobia about this that I felt uncertain about what I was feeling. My imagination led me to believe that there was not just one lump lurking in there but hundreds in each breast. Dr Bradbury kindly agreed to examine me himself every three months.

I remember those visits only too well. The doctor wore his spectacles on the end of his nose and would look over them. I would stand there petrified at what he might find. Every time his hand paused during the examination I would say, 'What's the matter?' To which he responded, 'Nothing, I'm just concentrating', and I would say, 'Well, don't. You're scaring me to death!' The relief was enormous, sheer ecstasy at having survived a further three months. I very soon wondered, though, which occasion would be the one where I was told, 'Oh, I think we had better get this checked out.' The uncertainty became unbearable, especially for a control freak like me who liked, in truth *needed*, to be in charge of her own destiny.

* * *

Ever since Mum died, breast cancer was my dread. Despite all the doctors' reassurances to the contrary, I had always thought that this must be hereditary. I knew of so many women who had developed breast cancer and ultimately suffered the same fate as my mum. How could I not be scared? Now, suddenly, I was thrown into a world I had feared for so long. I knew now that breast cancer could be hereditary; yet kindly, well-meaning GPs had dismissed this out of hand. I didn't want to wait until I got the wretched disease. I wanted to discover a means of preventing it. Although I actually had a nice figure, I took no pleasure from my breasts. They were just the very enemy that could kill me, ticking time bombs just waiting to get me. Yet I was calm and rational about it all. I understood the fear and I understood that I should not become neurotic. At the same time, however, I felt I had been given an opportunity to find a solution during this window of time, and work out how to beat this life-threatening problem.

I heard an item on the Jimmy Young radio programme one day about Tamoxifen, a drug that was being trialled to prevent breast cancer. Of course, with my usual impatience I charged back to the ever patient Doctor Bradbury, telling him all about the Jimmy Young programme and this new drug. He promised to write off somewhere for me, in order to establish the availability of this trial and my eligibility.

When I heard no more, I once again booked an appointment and was told that this Tamoxifen drug would *not* be suitable for someone of my age. It was a trial, therefore I might only get the placebo, but also the side effects were not helpful. I was told it could bring on a whole catalogue of uncomfortable issues with no guarantees either. In any event, I could not be part of this.

My sister Diane came to stay one weekend, and we went for a walk through the beautiful Lathkildale. We chatted endlessly about the latest turn in events over this whole breast cancer issue. Like me, Diane had been worrying, but we had not particularly vocalised our fears to each other before. I had no idea that she, too, had fretted over the years as I had done.

I remember the exact location where I quipped that I had a good mind to have surgery now before developing the breast cancer; after all, if it was so important to catch it early, this would be the best possible time. I said it as a joke, but in reality that was the eureka moment. Of course, it didn't appear that way at the time; it was more a flippant remark, but over the next few weeks I explored the prospect in my own head. What was I really scared of about breast cancer?

Was it the surgery?

No.

Was it treatment?

Partly. I think I was more concerned about losing my long blonde hair than my breasts.

Was it the prospect of dying at a young age like my mother?

Most definitely.

And so my own counselling was done inwardly. I am totally realistic, and felt that this was the obvious solution. Unless someone could convince me of a treatment that was guaranteed to work, then how could I ignore my own brainwave? I had already mused on the possibility of low-dose chemotherapy as a pre-emptive measure that would, hopefully, mop up any initial cancer cells. This seemed to everyone a long shot at that time. I was hardly likely to persuade someone to invent this especially for me, right now.

I discussed the whole issue with Chris, who was totally supportive. He said he would rather have me alive without breasts, than dead with them. He was calm and logical, and it never occurred to me that he would be anything other. I asked if he felt it would make a difference to him, but he strongly denied that. He, like me, was glad to have found a way round this. We were neither of us emotional about the decision at all. I was really quite pleased to have the ingenuity to come up with a solution to a seemingly insuperable problem. It may have seemed radical, but the inevitability of breast cancer seemed too obvious and frightening to deal with in any other way.

I was referred to my local hospital in Buxton to see breast surgeon Peter England. He had already seen the notes from my doctor and was totally bemused. He was very frank with me.

He said, 'This is a request I could never have envisaged. Most women are pleading with me to preserve their breast tissue.'

But he did concede that there was a way of thinking now that, in some families, breast cancer could possibly be hereditary, and that a clinic was being formed in Manchester under geneticist Gareth Evans. He told me they were 'crying out' for families like mine with multiple breast cancers to aid research into locating the gene or genes responsible. He then said that if I would agree to go there, and if they thought it appropriate, he would gladly perform this operation. Of course, I readily accepted.

I was sent forms to fill in about my family. I had all the information readily to hand, thanks to our earlier detective work, and supplied all the details. The day of the appointment arrived, Chris came with me. I wanted to present my case in a well-conceived fashion, and not be dismissed as a neurotic female. Gareth Evans was a young, enthusiastic doctor, avid for research, and we got on famously from the start.

He explained that they were currently researching the possibility of two genes being responsible for breast cancer in some families, BRCA1 and 2. He thought that in our family it was likely to be BRCA1, as this gene typically conferred occasional risk of ovarian cancer, which had affected two of my relatives. He was keen for our family to join a research study, and to donate blood to assist in the detection and sequencing of this gene. We were obviously delighted to help in any way possible.

Gareth explained that a fault in either of these genes signified an 80-90 per cent risk of developing breast cancer. He also said that I had a 50:50 chance of inheriting the fault from my mother, and therefore estimated my current breast cancer risk at 40-45 per cent. He said that my proposals for surgery were reasonable, given this dreadful family history, but also enquired how I would feel if – say in two years' time – a genetic test was developed, and I was found *not* to carry the fault?

My response to this question was very speedy – it didn't matter. Whatever the result of a future test, or whenever that might be, he couldn't possibly give me any bad news. If I carried the 'fault', well, I would have done the right thing; if I was found *not* to carry the fault, that would be excellent news, too, as I wouldn't then be able to pass it on to my daughter. Gareth agreed that yes, indeed, that was the bottom line. He could tell that my mind was made up, clearly and driven by pure reason. He said he would write to Peter England, confirming that the surgery was the right course of action for me.

I sat outside Gareth's office, waiting to be taken for a thorough check and a mammogram. The door was slightly ajar, and I overheard Gareth's dictation to Mr England approving the surgery. To this day, I can still hear the words 'quite honestly, I don't blame her', which, to me, meant they were more than just going along with me; they were a professional and personal endorsement of my own conclusions. As far as I knew, no one else had ever opted to have a mastectomy for *preventative* reasons. It seemed I was probably going to be the first person in the UK to take these steps. It seemed clear that this would be possibly the first preventative mastectomy in the country.

I was bright enough to realise that for something as pioneering as this situation was, the medical team had to be sure I had no doubts. We live in times of litigation, and I wanted people to feel comfortable that my request was well conceived and non-hysterical, and that after the operation I would not suddenly turn into some idiot wanting to sue them for agreeing to fulfil my own wishes. My chief concern was that my request for surgery would be refused, because I knew that the medical people who were co-operating with me to perform this procedure were taking a risk. I was asking them to fly in the face of current practice, which assuaged vanity, and sought to allow women to retain their breasts at all costs, if safely possible.

Fortunately, Gareth Evans is extremely perceptive. He is tremendously easy to converse with and views his patients as intelligent beings who, although they may not have a medical background, are nevertheless smart enough to work things out. He is now one of the world's most respected and well-liked geneticists in the field of hereditary breast cancer and neurofibromatosis.

A further appointment was soon arranged to see Peter England. This time the atmosphere of our meeting, and Mr England's attitude, were very different.

Mr England looked me straight in the eye and said, 'Well, they're coming off then, I gather.'

Even I, with my strongly pragmatic nature, was slightly taken aback by his blunt phraseology, but nevertheless I gamely agreed. He asked me when I would like the operation.

I thought for only a few seconds. 'Well, the cows go out to pasture around the middle of April, and we start silaging in June, so towards the end of April would be perfect.' He grinned, and said he had never scheduled an operation around a herd of cows before!

Having now got over the hurdle of convincing the medical profession of my reasoning and sanity, I now had the task of explaining the situation to others – friends, family and acquaintances.

Everyone I told outside my close family listened in horror to my proposals. 'Isn't that a bit drastic?' were the exact words uttered by the majority. I found that I needed to take at least half an hour to explain my decision, to describe the severity of the problem and my family background. I explained the fact that, given the poor outcomes of some of the treatments, and the likelihood of developing the disease and needing surgery anyway at some point, this seemed the most logical thing to do. To undergo surgery prior to developing the disease was the way to avert needless chemotherapy and death. To me, it was as stark and blindingly obvious as that.

Given sufficient time to assimilate the facts, most people began to understand my thinking. Nearly all declared they thought I was extremely brave, for which I could take no credit. I knew I was not brave enough to cope with cancer. I merely thought I was resourceful enough to have figured out a way to deal with all of this. I found though, as the time for surgery came ever closer, and needing to tell more and more people, I just said that I was going into hospital to have the bit removed where breast cancer starts. It wasn't completely honest, but it made them feel better.

Then, as the operation drew near, the collywobbles started. Not from any concern over this being the correct decision – of that I had no doubt whatsoever – but from anxiety over actually putting oneself through surgery. The attendant risks of anaesthetics, blood clots, etc. weighed on my mind, but I was never going to back out. It was rather like going to the dentist. You don't want to go, but you do go nevertheless. In the dark hours, I thought through things in my usual practical way. The surgery seemed inevitable – almost. Dying wasn't. The surgery was not of the invasive kind: nothing like open-heart surgery or suchlike. Yes, no problems there. I was fit and well at the moment; in optimum health from looking after 350 animals. Now was absolutely the right time for me . . . And so I counselled myself through this difficult period.

But I was still scared. Who wouldn't be?

I went into hospital on 20 April 1992. The operation was scheduled for the following morning. Peter England had worked wonders with his operating list, co-ordinating his holidays and my cattle. My friend

Linda (not to be confused with Linda, my friend since childhood) came to see me the evening before the operation. She was my walking companion, very caring but with an extremely dry sense of humour. Just the person I needed to chat to that evening. Perfect.

The following day I remember only as a blur, caused by that marvellous invention, the pre-med pill. It worked like a dream. I fell asleep and woke up later, wondering when I would be going down for the operation. I asked Chris and he told me I had already been. I think I was so full of morphine I just wasn't with it.

But the relief was amazing. I felt the most privileged person in the world. Here was I in a ward with 29 other women, all of whom were waiting to learn the results of their operations; waiting to have further scans. Was the lump in their breast cancerous? Would they need chemotherapy? Had the cancer spread? What was the prognosis?

Lucky, *lucky* me – I had just two scars. No need for any further investigations. Game over. The elation was incredible. I had survived.

I had undergone a total, complete double mastectomy, and the surgeon told me he had been careful to remove as near as possible 100 per cent of my breast tissue. In a sense, the operation was simple enough. Non-invasive, leaving just two straight scars. This was exactly as I expected. I had not opted for immediate reconstruction. Mr England, my surgeon, felt that he could make a better job of reconstruction after, say, six months. I had not opted to keep my nipples, since the operation was all about removing as much breast tissue as possible. I had said goodbye to my breasts. It was a choice I was comfortable with.

I felt the sacrifice was minute compared with the alternative. I had sacrificed a part of my body in order to keep it all.

Two drains were inserted in each side. These were essentially coiled tubes, ending in removable bags, that enabled the liquid to simply drain away. The nurse suggested I had carrier bags to put them in when moving around. Chris had duly brought along two Co-op carrier bags, but I felt that being possibly the first person to undergo this procedure I should merit at least Harrods bags to give a touch of class! He compromised the next day and found some similar green ones we had – from John Lewis, I think.

The scars were simple and neat, almost meeting in the middle. It was no worse than I had expected; better in fact. To be honest, they were the least of my worries. I had survived the operation and cheated this ghastly disease. I wanted to *celebrate* the departure of my breasts, not mourn their loss. I was told I would probably be in hospital for a week to 10 days, until the drains could be removed safely, the scars were healed and the stitches removed. Now *that* was something to look forward to! I did rather dread that without a general anaesthetic.

I thought about how Chris would react to what he would see. Indeed, I wondered, how *did* you show a husband? Just how do you approach this? I needn't have fretted at all. The following day, when Chris visited me, he brought the customary bottle of Lucozade, which he promptly spilt all over me and the bed. The nurses took on the task of changing the bed and asked Chris to go with me to the bathroom to help me change out of my now extremely sticky, orange-stained nightdress. Well, that at least solved that little quandary! Chris made no comment other than to agree how neat it all was.

The next few days in hospital had their amusing moments. I was high as a kite to be honest. I had made great friends with Lynn, the girl in the next bed, who had also had a total mastectomy and had been told that all the lymph nodes were clear. She was, of course, elated, and the two of us were like naughty school children. I had a whale of a time. One poor lady had a dreadful reaction to the drugs she had been given and was running amok in the ward, hallucinating like crazy. I found her sitting under my bed begging me to help her mend her boat. She was inconsolable. Eventually I decided it might be best to go along with this, so I heaved myself, drains and all, from my lovely comfy bed and crawled under it ostensibly to help her. A nurse soon came along and surveyed the scene. She was used to the antics of the other lady, but asked me, 'What are you doing?'

'Mending her boat!' I replied. What other answer was there?

And so our next few days progressed in that same vein of euphoria. That's how it was; a wonderful feeling. I doubt I will ever again feel such relief.

The nurses, doctors, and other patients kept telling me how brave I was. I really didn't feel I deserved the compliment. I kept denying this, saying I had done what I'd done because I wasn't brave enough to face the alternative. It was everyone else in the ward that was brave. How they coped with their fear was incredible to me. So many ladies waiting for scans each day, discussing their future treatments. I had none of this. I was so, so lucky, that's all.

The pain killers I was taking caused a problem though – one not usually discussed anywhere but in a hospital. As the saying goes 'pride goes out the window'. The nurse wrote down on my sheet 'bunged up to the eyeballs'. Each time the doctor did his rounds, the concern would focus on my lack of going to the toilet. Eventually everyone was asking, 'Have you been yet?' It became a standing joke in the ward.

My lovely family, Diane, Dad and Olive, travelled several times from Leicester to Manchester to visit me. Becky came most days with Chris. I wanted desperately for her to see me fit and looking well, especially as I was conscious that this could well be something she might have to consider in the future. This wasn't hard to achieve. The immense adrenalin rush I was experiencing made me look and feel fantastic. Every day more flowers would arrive. Lindsay, who worked as a researcher with Dr Gareth Evans had collected some of the breast tissue for research purposes. She was there when the doctor told me that the lab had thoroughly examined all the tissue removed and had confirmed it was completely clear of cancer. It doesn't get any better than that.

After nine days I was discharged. I was both glad and sorry as one very quickly becomes institutionalised in these places. I had made dozens of brilliant friends, and they had been my saviours. This place had enabled me to move forward in my life with an attitude I had not had for 20 years. I now had a real expectation of living beyond 40. Many people said to me, 'You could do this then get run over by a bus.' Well, I guess that's right, but wouldn't I try to move out of the bus's way? So, leaving the hospital was not done without very fond farewells. Olive came to the farm to stay and look after me for a few days. Her cooking was up to its usual standard and was infinitely preferable to the hospital food. Though I didn't really have complaints in that department. You cannot expect gourmet meals served from a trolley, and I think they do brilliantly to manage to offer the choices they do.

Due to the increased risk of ovarian cancer associated with the BRCA genes, and also evident in my family's history, I was to attend for an ovarian scan the following week. I wasn't unduly worried about this, but was terrified by the findings. The scan showed a cyst, relatively small as yet, and with no clear indication as to what it might be. The consultant suggested this might just be a follicle cyst, which would disappear at a different part in my cycle. I was to wait six weeks, then return for a further scan.

This was awful. Gone was my earlier elation at pulling off the 'breast cancer prevention' feat. Something else was out to get me that I had made no plans for. I waited the six weeks with a sick dread, fearing the worst while hoping for the best.

I concentrated on repairing myself from the surgery I had just undergone. There were exercises to be performed regularly. These were simple enough, more or less gentle stretching movements with my arms in different directions to ensure that, in the healing process, the skin didn't tighten too greatly.

My mind was confused as to what had actually happened to the tissue. It was a strange sensation, losing a part of yourself and grappling with how one part of the body now joined up with another. As I ran my hand down my chest it was the oddest feeling to suddenly go from one part of my body immediately to another part that felt unconnected, yet now was. I cannot really explain it, except to say that it is incredibly odd. It didn't bother me though, and was really quite intriguing – experimenting to get a clearer understanding myself. I was happy with my new body shape.

When I left the hospital, I was given two very soft pads to put into my bra. Of course, I could now choose exactly which cup size I would like to be – no need whatsoever to stick with the originals. As it happens, I didn't dislike my breast size at all. If anything, I was happier to go smaller.

The format for this was to wear the soft ones for around six weeks, then return to the hospital for the jelly-like ones to replace them. I had no idea though just what antics these things would cause.

A week or so after coming home, a friend took me down to Bakewell, and we went for tea in one of the numerous cafes in the town. I was wearing a button-up, V- neck blouse, fairly low cut. As I leaned across the table to reach for the enormous teapot to pour another cup, one of the silly little pads chose that moment to slide upwards out of the top of my bra. It was obviously responding to the pressure from my arm – but it didn't slide back down again.

My friend Margaret and I both burst out laughing, and I dashed to the ladies to push the offending article back in place. Sadly, I had been too lazy to start sewing pockets into my bras. Sewing is not my thing unfortunately. Over the next couple of years, these items took on a life of their own, popping out at the most inopportune moments. But it was so difficult to predict when.

When I returned to the hospital for the second scan, the head of department, an obviously knowledgeable lady, performed the scan and interpreted the results. She was extremely frank. She said the cyst was still there, but only about two centimetres and it didn't look sinister. However, given my family history, she thought it might be better to get the ovary removed to be on the safe side.

I didn't need telling twice. I rang Gareth from my mobile and managed to get an appointment in record time. Ten minutes to be precise!

Gareth was very accommodating. He'd already received a call from the radiographer, and saw me right away although he hadn't got a clinic. 'Sod's Law' sprang to mind as we discussed this latest development. I said, 'Look, while I'm asleep just do a full hysterectomy. Get rid of those bits that obviously aren't any further use to me, and can only potentially be a further cancer threat. I'm not planning any more children, and now I haven't any breast tissue, I'm not at increased risk of breast cancer. I can have HRT – in fact, I'll have the biggest HRT implant you can find!'

Having a hysterectomy would bring about immediate and early menopause, but having HRT would prevent this. In women who undergo a simple oophrectomy (just the ovaries removed) the HRT needs to be a combination of oestrogen and progesterone. With a full hysterectomy, oestrogen only can be taken. Trials have shown that HRT can very slightly increase the risk of developing breast cancer, however, the oestrogen only does not increase the risk so significantly, and in any case I had no breast tissue. Although it has these side effects, HRT has a brilliant reputation for making you feel good, and for boosting energy. I can now definitely agree with that.

Gareth understood my humour, my own personal

way of dealing with all of this, and arranged for me to see Dr Donnai. He was fabulous, a really humane surgeon, who scheduled my appointment for a full hysterectomy immediately.

So, within only eight weeks of my double mastectomy, I underwent a full hysterectomy. The operation went smoothly, although I found it more painful afterwards than the mastectomy had been. The registrar was clearly in on the joke of the giant HRT implant. When he came to see me after the surgery, he looked at my scars. He pointed to the hysterectomy scar and said wryly, 'You think that's your hysterectomy, don't you?' I nodded and he shook his head. He pointed at the smaller half-inch scar and dryly said, 'That's your hysterectomy – the bigger one is your HRT implant!'

As it happens, I had endless things wrong with me evidently – fibroids, endometriosis, but *no* cancer. In the end, it was just what is known as a follicle cyst.

Oh joy, oh joy, and thank God!

Although I was fatigued from two major operations in less than two months, I was determined to get back to life properly. The first shower I took in hospital induced a virtual collapse. Talk about weak! The wonderful big, strong nurse who was caring for me, wrapped me in my towel and held me up, pressing me against her own body. It was an extremely strange sensation for me to be utterly worn out through taking a shower. She practically carried me back to bed in an exhausted condition, where I collapsed into the mountain of fluffy pillows, feeling totally blissful at the extraordinary comfort of a hospital bed.

Life took off again. Six weeks after my operations, I was back on stage, involved in my favourite hobby

– musical theatre. I was taking part in *South Pacific* at the Buxton Opera House, singing, dancing and laughing again.

My stamina from working full time on the farm had merely been dented from the traumas of the past two months, not totally crushed. Along with the satisfaction of cheating cancer, I began to feel an elation I had never experienced before. It was fantastic! How much of it was natural adrenaline, relief and joy, and how much the benefits of HRT is hard to say, but nevertheless I now had a zest for life I had not experienced in a long while. There was nothing I felt that I couldn't achieve.

I returned to hospital for my six-month check-up and to arrange for my breast reconstruction. Mr England was very pleased with my progress in every way. It was clearly a relief to him that I had coped exactly as I had believed I would. He had put himself on the line here – relying on my own common-sense approach and Gareth's professional backing.

We discussed the reconstruction, but at this stage I had no idea what 'size' I wanted to be. I was thus packed off home with three different cup sizes to try out and get used to, with the opportunity of a further appointment later. This was to no avail either, as my young daughter Becky just loved borrowing these falsies to stuff up her jumper and parade around. Actually finding a pair to put on to go out anywhere became impossible. Becky's bedroom, at the best of times, resembled an untidy skip. The prospect of finding a matching pair of these things hardly existed. I would find an odd pair – or two 'right' ones, but never the pairing I needed, so very often I would just not bother.

One particularly funny event with these unmanageable items happened during the show *Calamity Jane*. I took the lead part for Belper Operatic Society. This role demanded Calamity to get undressed in a temper, showing her annoyance with Wild Bill Hickok by stalking around the stage chucking off clothes just down to bloomers and a camisole top. One night disaster struck. As I pulled the dress over my head, one of the special jelly-type prostheses I was wearing fell out onto the floor with a noticeable splat. I looked at Bill who, quick as a flash, remarked to a mirthful audience that he didn't know whether to stamp on it or shoot it! And so the laughs continued, and as usual my sense of humour was my most useful armour.

BRINGING BRCA TO THE WORLD

Gareth Evans and his team were working hard with all the blood samples that had been provided by my extended family. I was, as usual, thirsty for knowledge and information. Gareth sent me various teaching modules used by medical students moving into the field of genetics. I studied these avidly, determined to understand the whole DNA structure – what a gene was and how it functioned. What rapidly became apparent was that my family was in no way unique, but thanks to our excellent investigative work it had become obvious that a risk existed for us and we were in this group of 'gene fault carriers'.

I soon learned that, with all the high-risk genes, around one in 200 women carry a fault in one of them. The actual genes had not yet been fully sequenced, so testing was still not really possible, although the discovery that at least two genes were responsible for the majority of the 'high risk' cases was being intensively worked on around the world, in collaboration with other scientists. BRCA1 was located on Chromosome 17, BRCA2 on Chromosome 13. Those two genes were likely to be responsible for about half of the very high-risk faults, in other words one in 400 would carry a fault in one of these two genes. In the future, maybe a couple of years later, research would determine several more genes, a fault in which would confer a higher than average risk of developing breast cancer.

This led me to a feeling of responsibility. I was experiencing relief and excitement in life that I had suppressed subconsciously. I wasn't aware of it at the time, but since the surgery I had been living on a constant high. I was wise enough to realise that my course of action would not suit everyone, but I believed that people should at least be made aware that breast cancer can be inherited; that there were things one could do about it, that the surgical option was viable and acceptable. It was not the hideous, macabre procedure that many had tried to portray, but a lifesaver.

The facts are fairly straightforward. Most people develop breast cancer by chance. These chances could be linked to lifestyle, breast density, environmental factors, or combinations of genes that give some increased risk of developing breast cancer in your life-time. The few high-risk gene carriers can be screened regularly or opt for surgery. Screening can be carried out by MRI in some instances, particularly if the fault is in BRCA1; the type of breast cancer typical in these cases is more difficult to detect through mammograms alone. Mammography, however, is a useful addition and, provided people realise that the screening does not *prevent* breast cancer but aims to detect it as early as possible, then for some this will be the preferred option. To adopt a watchful, waiting approach. For those who want to be more proactive, but don't wish to take the surgical route, there are various drugs trials that are already showing some degree of success. The Tamoxifen trial early figures denoted a potential 50 per cent reduction in risk.

Having an oophrectomy before the age of 40 is also thought to significantly reduce the risk in known gene carriers from a lifetime risk of 80-85 per cent down to around half that. The studies that have been performed on those women opting for the mastectomy choice have all shown at least a 90 per cent reduction in risk.

In some families, there is an increased risk of developing ovarian cancer. It seems to vary from family to family, but in general the risk given with a fault is 20-60 per cent lifetime risk.

Men with the BRCA2 fault also have some increased risk of developing breast cancer, in addition to a risk of developing prostate cancer. The IMPACT study run by the Royal Marsden Hospital and Cancer Research UK is looking into these very risks in men. It will be a lifelong job for me to raise awareness that the gene can be passed down through the male line since, even today, many GPs don't realise this. In fact, half of these faults will be inherited from the father, but this won't be detected since nothing will be evident.

I felt it was my duty to share my positive situation with others – but how? A distinct reticence overtook me as to how the media might seize on this. I wanted someone to tell the story exactly as it was, not some sensationalised over-dramatised cheap story, but an intelligent factual piece.

I chose to tell my story to the *Independent* newspaper. They were slightly bemused by my phone call, but sent a journalist to interview me and write a story. The lady who met me was delightful, an excellent listener, and related the story in the exact way I had hoped for. I realised this would have an effect, but was totally unprepared for the intensity of the media interest.

The Big Breakfast was a popular morning TV programme. They pestered and pestered Becky and me to go on as guests. Becky, who was about 12 at the time, was determined we should go, thinking how exciting that would be. Eventually I allowed myself to be talked into it.

It was all a very unusual experience. A big chauffeur-driven limo picked us up from the station and delivered us to a swish hotel. The next morning, a similarly glamorous car arrived to take us to the Big Breakfast House. When the interviews were over, a car of a far lesser elegance and statement arrived to deliver us back to the train station.

The interview went well. I remember Gaby Roslin saying they had contacted the Royal Marsden Hospital who apparently stated there was no evidence of any genes relating to breast cancer.

'What?' I exclaimed in reply. 'Who did you speak to? The cleaner?' The camera crew were by this time rolling around with laughter.

This exploit and others gave rise to a series of nonsensical magazine articles which were written exactly in the style I had tried so hard to avoid. After this little foray into the media, although glad to have brought things into the open and raised awareness, I became reticent about any further dealings with them.

Gareth brought a proposition to me. A documentary called *The Decision*, a series of six life-changing and thought-provoking documentaries had been commissioned by Channel 4. They were intrigued by the whole issue of my experience and I was invited to meet the producer, Sally Dixon, to see if I would be happy to be the subject of one episode. Sally came to the farm to see me, and I immediately loved her great sense of humour and sensible take on my story. She wanted me to be comfortable with the whole experience, and for the most part I was happy.

Filming started in 1994 and followed many strands of our investigations. I really wanted to find out the full extent of the breast cancers in our wider family. Jennifer said she thought our mothers had another cousin, Jean Farnsworth, who was Grandma's brother's granddaughter. She had lived in Brighton but had been buried in the family cemetery, Wirksworth, having died at the age of 57. I sent for her death certificate, which was a relatively easy thing to do.

When I opened the envelope and unfolded the neat new certificate, cause of death was as expected – 'carcinomatosis of the right breast'. In other words, yet another breast cancer, this time inherited through many generations on the male side of the family. My grandmother was one of eight brothers and sisters; Jean was the granddaughter of the eldest brother, Tom. I was later to discover that my grandmother and her brothers and sisters had inherited the gene fault from their father's side of the family. I scoured the certificate for any other information it might provide. The death had been registered by Laurence Farnsworth, Jean's husband, and gave his occupation as college principal.

I guessed Laurence Farnsworth would be retired by now, but I nevertheless set about contacting all the colleges in and around Brighton. I did eventually find where he had worked, left my details, and asked if they could possibly contact him. This they did, and later that afternoon I received a call from him. Laurence Farnsworth was an elderly gentleman, but clearly well-educated and still completely in control of everything. I tentatively explained who I was and my reason for contacting him. I knew his wife had died from breast cancer, I said, and I explained the relationship with the rest of our family. Most importantly of all, I asked whether he had any children.

He took this all in, accepting it calmly. And yes, indeed, he had a daughter, Vanessa, who was 42 years old. At this, I felt I had given him more than enough information for the time being.

Laurence rang me back later to say that, of course, Vanessa must be informed of the family history. He would never forgive himself if something happened to her without prior warning. Later that evening I received a call from Vanessa. I think she was in total shock. Suddenly, from having a very common involvement with breast cancer – her 57-year-old mother the only family member to have contracted the disease – she now found herself with a pile of relatives she didn't know, harbouring some absolutely awful news.

The Decision programme followed this meeting in depth, the subsequent genetic tests performed on all of our family, and Vanessa's eventual surgery. Vanessa had been adamant that she could *never* consider the elective surgery route that I had taken. All the way through the programme the theme never changed. I was pragmatic about my own choice but felt it was up to Vanessa to make her own decisions. Incredibly, within only minutes of receiving her genetic test results, which confirmed she had indeed inherited the fault, Vanessa was proclaiming that surgery was the obvious choice. On film she had argued the point with her husband. Okay, it might not happen for years, so what is the point in spending all of this time being worried? Towards the end she even stated, 'Well, it's no great shakes really!' The film followed her through all these processes, and her surgery. Sally Dixon had done an excellent job for Windfall Films and Channel 4.

Meanwhile I was getting on with life. I founded Peak Performance, a theatre company based in the Peak District, to put on shows at the Buxton Opera House, and raise positive awareness of hereditary breast cancer. I was absolutely determined that no one should perceive me as some wilting violet who had abused her body. Moreover, I wanted people to see the zest for life I had now found, the liberation I felt, and my commitment to informing others about this hideous disease and its familial effects. To face it in this way was an acceptable option. Obviously I wasn't expecting everyone to go charging around demanding surgery; of course not. That would be highly inappropriate. But I felt it was terribly important to make people realise that there were acceptable options which could help save lives.

I took on more musical theatre roles, while working like mad on the farm to try to make ends meet. Unfortunately, the 15.4 per cent interest rates were crippling. We reluctantly left the farm and bought a lease on Moorhall Post Office. It was not only a post office but also an off-licence and newsagent, general store and fresh bakery, selling hot and cold sandwiches. Oh my goodness! How would we keep on top of *this* lot, with Chris still busy working in the police force? This was another silly time for us.

The mornings started at five-thirty a.m. when my spiteful alarm clock woke me up with its relentless noise. I would leap out of bed, run downstairs, and set up the outside market stall of fruit and vegetables. The next task was to bring in the stacks of newspapers, mark them up for the paper lads, and when the first staff arrived an hour later, set out for Sheffield cash-and-carry. After running round spending £1,000 on stock, I returned as fast as possible to unload the van and get ready to open the post office section of the shop at nine a.m. Gosh, it felt like an entire day's work before I even started with that.

When the post office closed, I had to balance the books and spend a further two hours on duty in the off-licence and grocery section. Oh, for the farm and 350 cattle, how much easier! But I did have staff, and it was a friendly shop where the locals from the estate called in regularly. One old lady, Beryl, would visit every day, and sit on her special stool at the end of the counter. For some reason she had really taken to me. I didn't – and couldn't – foresee then what a major part Beryl would play in many people's lives in the future.

My hobby, walking, suffered from being at the shop. I liked nothing better than to set out with a map of the Peak District and find a footpath I didn't know. Linda, my walking companion from the farm days, wanted to go on a walking holiday, so I tagged a few days onto August Bank Holiday and devised a route. We were dropped off just outside Halifax and walked home, stopping at bed and breakfast venues on the way, a 70-mile journey.

Our first couple of stops were fairly unremarkable,

but on the third morning I woke up and my legs just would not go. Well, Linda and I laughed and laughed; I had a hot bath and coaxed them into action. We set out in the misty weather with our midday sandwiches packed into our rucksacks. This particular part of the journey involved crossing the moors for about five miles. It wasn't long before a thick mist descended and we were truly lost. Eventually the mist lifted slightly and I was able to verify that, yes, we had been walking in the right direction. Hallelujah. In fact, we were only around half a mile from our next B&B, The Strines Hotel, a fifteenth-century coaching house. At around half past three we had 'reached our destination', to quote Tom Tom. Thank heavens.

Yes, a room was available, but all their rooms had four-poster beds. By this time I couldn't have cared less, I would have slept in a cowshed like Mary and Joseph if necessary. We sat downstairs in the bar and had an enormous pot of tea. After about five cups each, we were told our room was ready, but my legs had seized up yet again. I somehow made it up the stairs and got into the gorgeous old-fashioned room, with its gynormous four-poster bed. But no way could I climb into it, I was stiff as a board. Linda gave me a hump up, and I ended up flat on my back, sinking into the feather mattress and taking Linda with me. Just exactly at that point, the staff chose to bring a tray up to the room, noted the shenanigans and apologised for interrupting!

'It's fine, come in!' I insisted, mortified at the girl's impression. I could just imagine her going back downstairs to the owners, who had surveyed us suspiciously from the start. Well, of course, you just had to see the funny side. I have never been back there since!

Another amusing story happened at the post office

and concerned my silicone breast prostheses. They were forever popping out of my bra and I got used to finding them in odd places. Quite often, as I lugged around the sacks of potatoes and trays of fruit and vegetables, these little blighters would often turn up in those potato sacks or vegetable trays, having disappeared unnoticed earlier in the haste of rushing round.

I remember a particularly uncomfortable moment, though, when the Post Office Auditor came to audit the books and check the safe. Although the shop was called Moorhall Post Office, the post office section was actually really tiny. A little one-man cubicle, complete with night safe. Definitely not enough room for two. The auditor turned up before we opened, which was the usual procedure. He had a big, old-fashioned briefcase which he brought into this cubicle with him. He requested that I empty the contents of the safe for him to check and verify as part of this audit. I duly got down on my hands and knees, vying for space with another body, and his briefcase. There was scarcely enough space to open the safe door at the best of times!

I left him with the money and stamps, and got on with the usual routine of dealing with customers, but a few minutes later one of my assistants pointed at me and said, 'You've lost one again.' I looked down, and lo and behold I had indeed lost one. This was a regular event and even our customers had been known to help in the search! After exhausting all the usual places, it suddenly occurred to me that the post office might just be where the offending object was hiding. The auditor was busy counting stamps and money, and saw me hovering around peering inside the tiny booth. Eventually he asked if there was anything wrong.

Perhaps he thought I had some guilty secret; had purloined some of the post office stock or something. I shook my head – then spotted his briefcase. 'Nothing for it,' I thought, and summoned up the courage to ask to look inside it. That was tricky. I had no choice but to explain the situation to the astonished auditor, resulting in a really good laugh and he obligingly allowing me examine the interior of his case. I peered in, and there, nestling innocently, was the errant right breast. No use to him whatsoever, of course, and would have been a definite source of bafflement if he'd turned up at home with it. Now that *would* take some explaining!

Peak Performance took off. I had booked a week at Buxton Opera House, and had secured the performing rights to *My Fair Lady*. I used my amateur theatre contacts to bring together the best performers in the county. I soon stumbled on an excellent producer and musical director, who would cast the show for me. I inveigled Gareth Evans into auditioning for the lead – Professor Higgins – and I was delighted to be chosen to play Eliza Doolittle. I already had my Actors' Equity card and had taken several small parts in TV's *Peak Practice*, and had much musical theatre under my belt. We spent many hours in rehearsals for *My Fair Lady* – hard work, but a lot of fun.

The Decision had taken 18 months to complete, but the filming was generally a splendid time, spent with really nice people. And Sally, of course, as predicted, had been a delight to work with. The finished product was shown in February 1996. I was nervous before seeing the film – understandably, because so much of my private self had been poured into it. My intention had been that people should understand my thought processes, if my decisions were to have any value at all to others.

I needn't have worried. Sally had exactly and faithfully produced a perfect film of the events. As she said, little artistic licence was needed since, in truth, the story was compelling enough. During that 18 months of filming, two of the BRCA genes were discovered and a genetic test was developed for our family. Four of us took the test, and this was all filmed live. First of all, Jennifer's daughter, Helen, featured. She was only 21, but was found to have inherited the fault from her mum. I thought she came over brilliantly on the film. She was very pragmatic about the whole thing, so much so that when Gareth asked her how she felt, she answered that he had only told her what she already knew. She was unfazed and said that she would probably consider her options more carefully when she reached 30.

My sister Diane was found to be negative. She felt an overwhelming sense of guilt as she was the only one of us with a negative result. Of course, we were all very happy for her. It also gave hope too, that the 50:50 chance of inheriting the gene really did exist. Vanessa, whose story was filmed throughout, was found to carry the fault – as, of course, was I. Needless to say, in the run-up to the screening on Channel 4, the press office got to work on cranking the publicity machine up to full power. I was happy to oblige with umpteen interviews, which made the programme 'Pick of the Day' for many TV guides. It seemed there was a huge amount of interest in a process which had just, to me, seemed the only common-sense course of action.

The morning *The Decision* was due be aired, Helen

and I were invited onto *Good Morning with Anne and Nick* as the day's top story. The purpose, I supposed, was to show a trailer and advertise *The Decision*. Anne Diamond was off sick that day, so Nick was alone. As we waited for the live show to start, Nick was doing deep breathing exercises. Both Helen and I looked at each other. He appeared more nervous than we, which seemed crazy. Well, of course this just relaxed us further. Once on set, Nick asked the questions rather tentatively; clearly he felt concerns about raising this topic, and had no idea he was dealing with two people as relaxed as we were on this topic.

In the end, after a particular question, Helen and I were giggling away, and Nick just shook his head in disbelief.

He remarked to us, 'You have had to undergo this surgery voluntarily. Helen is calmly stating the same will happen to her one way or another, and you are both laughing about it.' He looked aghast, and this just made us giggle even more. Of course it made for great TV. There were no histrionics, no dramas; just an acceptance from us both that things could have been a whole heap worse.

The following day I received a massive number of calls, and the shop was a hive of activity in the days after the programme. People were clearly bowled over by the frankness of what they had watched.

One particular letter really caught at my heartstrings though. It was from a young girl named Andrea, and it was heartbreaking:

Dear Mrs Watson
I hope you don't mind me writing, but having watched you on The Decision, I felt that at last here was someone who would understand how I feel.

My mother developed breast cancer at age 27 and died aged 31. Her mother died at age 26 of the disease. I have tried to discuss the surgical option with a breast clinic, but they won't hear of it. Yet I have a little girl of two and a half and a little boy of one, and the thought of a third generation growing up motherless has always filled me with terror. I am now 25 and my sister is 27. The people we see in the clinic say that until there is a genetic test available they cannot act. But we have no living relative to be compared with ...

I rang Andrea immediately. I felt as if I was conversing with myself. She was sensible about her rationale, and completely at a loss as to why it should not appear logical to others. We got on so well and I promised to contact the breast unit on her behalf.

I rang and asked to speak with the head of the breast clinic. My aim was to explain, tactfully, the difference surgery had made to me, how I was now able to get on with life, and that as Andrea had come to her own conclusions here, it would surely be the appropriate course of action for her to do the same.

The doctor listened to what I had to say, but I was totally unprepared for his response:

'My dear, just because you have been on television does that mean you think you know more about my job than I do?'

I replied, 'Of course not, but I can totally understand how Andrea feels and thought you might find it useful to hear from someone who has actually gone through this; to hear at first hand the extreme elation and liberation I have experienced.'

My conversation with Andrea had been easy and I felt she ought to be given the opportunity to at least discuss this with himself or his colleagues. Far from being kind and understanding, he reverted to sarcasm and pomposity.

His parting shot to me was, 'My dear, you should be running my clinic for me.'

Oh dear, oh dear. Hopeless. Far from helping here, now we had a man backed into a corner; unlikely now to listen to reason for fear of losing face.

Clearly, a Plan B had to be set in action.

I approached Gareth and asked if Andrea and her sister could be seen at Manchester. This was a possibility, and he swiftly agreed. There were mechanisms in those days called 'extra-contractual referrals' for patients to be seen out of area.

The two girls were delighted. They booked, but while waiting for their initial appointment to come along, the proverbial axe dropped. They received a letter from their health authority stating that their out-of-area funding had been refused; the doctor himself had said that, in performing this operation without a test, perhaps only one of the girls might carry the faulty gene, in which case the other would have undergone an unnecessary operation.

Okay, yes, but which one? Applying his principles, the girls felt that *without* surgery, one of them might needlessly perish. The tide of relief which had buoyed them up for the past few weeks was swept away.

Andrea rang me with this devastating news. I immediately told her not to worry, I would sort it out. The challenge had arrived. What was the problem? I thought calmly and carefully over what had been refused . . . the service and the help? No, that had been easy enough to sort. It had been agreed. It was the finance. Well, we must organise this. How? No idea.

* * *

Pretty soon a master plan came to mind. I was a competent singer and I had a story to tell. So, along with the new story of the two girls' plight, why not release a record to raise the funds?

I immediately got onto several record labels to 'find a song'. I sent a recording I had already done of the Diana Ross song, 'When You Tell Me That You Love Me'. An extremely pleasant man from EMI told me he had a song which they were unlikely to use themselves, written by a girl called Ruth Graham, called 'Where Do I Go From Here?' He put us in touch with each other.

Ruth Graham was delighted and agreed that, given the appropriateness of the title, she could rewrite the words to the actual song to make them more relevant. I duly met Ruth down in Bedford, and we recorded the song. I had it copied several times, wrote the story of Andrea and her sister's plight, and sent it to several record labels.

Time dragged by and I was becoming increasingly despondent when a phone call came out of the blue one Friday afternoon while I was manning the post office. A young girl introduced herself as Louise from WH Smith, and said they had listened to the recording and would like to order . . . 3000 cassettes and 2000 CDs. Good grief! How does one act cool under those circumstances? I didn't. I showed exactly the enormous excitement I felt. It was impossible not to. All I had to do now was to get a record label. I continued down this line, and told HMV about the Smith order. Not to be outdone, they ordered too, but slightly fewer: only 1000 CDs and a mere 2000 tapes.

And then I suddenly realised that I didn't actually need a record label. If one wasn't forthcoming, well, the

CD was now sold. I had no intention of trying to become a major recording artist, so I set about acquiring my own record company. Friends jokingly said I should call it 'Dauntless' and so I did. Dauntless Records became a limited company. Within days the bar-coding was sorted, the manufacturing in progress and graphic design organised. In the inlay card, I wrote a piece aiming to raise awareness in a positive manner. I wanted to ensure that all those women affected by the fault gene should have access to *all* the options where appropriate, then full support, no matter what their choice: a mantra I have stuck by to this very day.

And so, Dauntless Records cut its first (and only) record. Its registered Head Office? A Walkers' crisp box in my kitchen!

I now realised that WH Smith and HMV had really placed their orders on the back of a potentially big story – which gave me an opportunity to raise even more positive awareness. Peak Performance's show was almost ready for its week of production, and now I had a record in the shops. I would defy anyone to think up a downbeat story with these two events.

Andrea and her sister Rhonda were sweet about sharing their story and helping to promote the single, but it became clear very quickly that we needed another 'hook'. Then a further eureka moment occurred. Why not hold a Hereditary Breast Cancer Awareness Week? The song could be the theme for the week, and the two girls' story a reason to promote the campaign. Perfect. The first problem, though, was how did one hold one of these days/weeks? Do you have to apply for them somewhere? I did a further round of ringing everyone in creation and found that no, apparently not. You just *say* it is, and then it *is* – provided you are up to the enormous task of sending a million press releases out to newspapers and so on with an appropriate story. Well, we had that all right!

The next job was to write a press release. I had no idea at all how those worked, so I just made it up as I went along. Luckily, Buxton Opera House had an excellent database and sent flyers out for us for *My Fair Lady*, leaving me with only the awareness week to publicise.

What I really needed, however, was a high-profile person to back the Awareness Week. Brilliant idea, I thought, and very easy to decide who to target. Why not start at the top? So I penned a letter to Diana, Princess of Wales.

Only a matter of days after this, I received a phone call from Diana's offices. They were checking the address in order to send me a letter.

The letter arrived.

Dear Wendy
It gives me great pleasure to be able to give you my
support and encouragement for National Hereditary
Breast Cancer Awareness Week. What could be more
important than to draw to the attention of everyone the
very real need to continue with all that still has to be done
in the research, diagnosis and treatment of cancer?
I have the deepest admiration for people like yourself
who have the strength of character to overcome all adver-
sity and who find the time and energy to devote yourselves
to such a worthwhile cause.
With my best wishes
Yours Sincerely
Diana

How amazing! I really could not believe it. I had not asked for compliments, just for Diana to put her name behind the Awareness Week.

The other important thing to do during the week, in addition to radio interviews, TV, etc. was to send a leaflet to every GP surgery in the country. If this informed the medical profession I was halfway there. Gareth helped to write the fact sheet and Ros Eeles, a respected geneticist from the Royal Marsden Hospital, came on board to help him. Between them, they sorted the details and we produced a simple A5 glossy flyer to send to the GP practices throughout the country. The information was given in a series of short bullet points on how to recognise hereditary breast cancer in families, to whom and where people should be referred, and a few details on the known identified genes BRCA1 and 2 and their attendant risk factors.

Then I set about posting 165,000 of these around the country. Gosh, what a task. But we did it, we managed. In fact, I had done such a good job of advertising this Awareness Week to come, that *Watchdog Healthcheck* rang me to ask if I knew about it, as they would like to film a piece about me to show during their week. Fantastic! I struck a hard deal with them. I would give them their interview, whatever they wanted. In return they must advertise my CD. This took a bit of bargaining, but I did it. They finished the clip with a long shot of the CD and a mention.

I worried that I had missed out something I could have capitalised on. WH Smith made the song their Record of the Week, which meant it was played in the stores, and a video shown; not your usual pop video but with photos and captions telling the story. Brian Stevens, musical editor for BBC Radio 2, playlisted the song. I was enormously grateful. I told him the story, and the fact that the Head Office of Dauntless Records Limited was in fact a Walkers' crisp box in my kitchen. He rose to the joke and said that if this took off I might be able to promote the office to the pantry!

And so National Hereditary Breast Cancer Awareness Week took place just two weeks after Peak Performance's debut show. Our production of *My Fair Lady* at Buxton Opera House that week hadn't been without its disasters. The saying that 'a bad dress rehearsal bodes well for a good opening' certainly holds true. In fact, a dress rehearsal more full of calamities is hard to envisage: the scenery and scenery plot we'd hired just did not work; the stage sofa collapsed; various cast members missed their cues.

Those were the days, and as always the disasters were the most memorable bit. So successful were the reviews, so great the spirit of those volunteering their time and skills in the bid to do something positive for hereditary breast cancer that Peak Performance became a regular institution, a permanent annual 'week' in the year-long calendar of events in the Opera House's busy schedule.

So, within a short time, somehow or other, I had managed to pull off two fairly big events, both successful in the end.

Gareth revealed to me that all our publicity efforts were having such an enormous effect that people were now coming to his clinic, and others. But genetics was not a field that was receiving any specialist funding, and it was up to each Health Authority to determine whether to fund these services or not. Some women could get nothing beyond Gareth's research money.

I soon took hold of this. For Gareth's clinic to be under threat was totally ridiculous, and unacceptable. How much money did it actually save? I visited a very amenable commissioner called Roy Dudley Southern at Manchester Health Authority, who listened to the story of my family. By now we had all been able to have a genetic test; three out of four of us as yet unaffected by breast cancer had tested positive for a fault in BRCA1; all had chosen to undergo preventive surgery.

Roy was a brilliant commissioner. He displayed empathy, along with a very professional approach to the business case I presented. Pretty soon I was being asked to visit several other Health Authorities by differ-ent geneticists. I went to Southampton, Nottingham, and more Health Authorities in the Manchester region. Each time it was successful, but was it really viable for me to go charging round the country getting individual Health Authorities to fund something? What would happen when the particular commissioner I dealt with was replaced by another?

It seemed to me I must do something on a wider scale. Gareth was still concerned over the fate of the clinic that he had built up. The wonderful work he was doing in the field of clinical research was now threatened; all due to the process of devolvement to the lowest level. Whose idea was this devolvement anyway?

I wanted to investigate the relative cost implications of treating breast cancer; the costs of treating tumours found earlier through screen detection as opposed to the do nothing, wait-and-see approach. Gareth introduced me to another wonderful man – Professor Michael Steele from St Andrews and Edinburgh University – who said he would help me with this research. The figures we found between us related to Denmark, but we soon made the relevant adjustments and I formatted them into a simple cost analysis table. I also used our family as a model. The results were obvious, the savings immense, and self-evident to non-medically trained people. Our idea would save money as well as lives.

Put simply, the cost of my surgery without reconstruction was £2,000; the cost with reconstruction, £4,000. The cost of a genetic test was £500 for the first test, then £30 for each subsequent test for other family members, once the fault or mutation had been located. The average cost of developing breast cancer undetected at the earliest stages, including for some hospice care, or just simply ongoing drug treatments, was reckoned to be £25,000 at that time. Detecting a cancer at the earliest stages could cut costs dramatically to around £5,000, even with long-term follow-up. Thus, it didn't take last year's *Mastermind* winner to work out the enormous savings. I concluded that genetic testing in our family had saved the NHS around £68,000.

Three of us had been found to carry the faulty gene; opting for elective surgery *before* developing cancer cost £10,000 in total. The genetic tests cost £620 for the four of us; £500 for the initial test in one of the 'affected' family members, and four simple tests at £30 each. In the three of us *with* the fault, our costs were £10,000 for the surgery. Yet if we had not had the surgery and (given our 80–90 per cent chances) gone on to develop the disease, possibly to the terminal stages, the costs would be nearer £75,000. Projected savings for the NHS of around £64,000; plus the fact that my sister Diane had been spared an unnecessary operation at a cost of £4,000; her £30 test had proved negative. Multiply this by the number of women at increased risk across Britain; surely it made sense to fund this type of health-care provision.

Of course, one always has to do battle with prevailing governments who are in it for the short term, their principle aim being to balance the books of the moment. However, I still thought the argument was persuasive.

I sent these findings to the then Health Minister, Stephen Dorrell. My own MP, Patrick Mcloughlin, made sure they found their way to him. BBC Health Correspondent Matt Youdale was making a further documentary, accompanied by myself, Gareth, and Professor Steele, and featuring an interview with Baroness Cumberlege, Minister for Women's Health. I was invited to meet her and was afraid that I would let everyone down. I was concerned that the clarity and purpose of my story may not be properly conveyed. I really did feel an enormous amount of responsibility.

I had no need to worry. Baroness Cumberlege was totally delightful. She was accompanied by a trio of civil servants, advising her and helping to take notes. We were invited into a high-ceilinged room with an enormous table and each offered a particular seat. Once I began with the précis of my story, recounting my personal relief and elation, and highlighting the difficulties others had encountered that had needed to be dealt with piecemeal, I was fine. She encouraged me, drawing the story from me. She already had a good grasp of what had been going on, where I was with everything, and she knew all about Princess Diana's involvement.

After listening thoughtfully to my story, Baroness Cumberlege asked me if I would set up an official helpline for people such as myself. She said the

Department of Health could give me a grant to do so. There was something known as 'Section 64 Grants' to enable novel projects and services such as this to work alongside the NHS. I was dumbfounded and didn't really quite understand to start with. My mission was to get genetic services funded; not start something myself. However, Baroness Cumberlege said that hearing me had a profound effect on her, and she told the BBC that she thought I would push this field forward in a way that the professionals perhaps couldn't.

This was her statement on the BBC documentary *Facing the Music*:

'I think she is enormously courageous and it is personal testimony. People like Wendy who, when they explain what the choices were for them and how they reached those choices, that has a profound impact on other women. I do congratulate her and I think she will move this whole area forward in a way that professionals can't.'

Naturally I agreed to this, and was excited at the endless possibilities. It would mean there would be an official reason to promote awareness. There really would be something for everyone who had been turned away. Geneticists Gareth and Ros readily agreed to be my advisors. How lucky was I to have people of their vast experience prepared to assist me. I needed to become either a registered charity, or align myself with one to act as host. My helpline became an 'arm of' such a body.

Once again, fate had taken a hand. In Manchester a new charity had just been founded called the Genesis Breast Cancer Prevention Appeal. This was a remarkable coincidence in timing and an even more remarkable charity. It was the vision of a group of surgeons and clinicians to build Europe's first breast cancer prevention centre. They wanted to provide a one-stop shop to cater for all the clinical needs of patients at increased 'familial risk' of breast cancer. Even more amazing, they all were intending to work free of charge. Fundraising efforts were devised with an emphasis on minimising costs. The Hereditary Breast Cancer Helpline would be a perfect partner. Genesis chairman, Lester Barr, has been a loyal supporter from the outset.

The plan was to have it all set up within six months. I continued to study genetics, hungry for any materials Gareth could send me. I read all the studies, researching everything I could on the subject so that I would be prepared for whatever anyone might throw at me. The one thing I had not completely considered was, how was I to find the time?

The solution came in a very strange way, as these things often do. One of my good friends, Beryl, who I had first met in the shop, had recently lost her husband. She was desperate for help or she would be forced to move into a care home. She begged our family to move in and stay with her so she could remain at home, quite rightly pointing out that this would be ideal for running the helpline. The house was perfectly laid out for this, as the only communal area needed was the kitchen. Beryl had her plan perfectly formulated. From her point of view there was nothing to think about. I would have the space and time to concentrate on the helpline. She would be allowed to remain at home with a little extra 'care'.

I was rather astonished at her request, and clearly needed to talk it through with Becky and Chris. We thought about it, and indeed it did seem a good plan.

Beryl's need was immense. She was desperate not to move, but I was reluctant to uproot hastily. Then, as time went on, Beryl's plight became more immediate. A spell in hospital forced the issue. She would not be allowed to return home without a carer, so we agreed to try it out. I placed the shop on the market, or should I say, someone approached us to buy it. The whole process seemed mapped out, as if ordained. We moved in, leaving solicitors to take care of all the financial arrangements.

Beryl, a devout Christian, told the vicar that she wanted to help in the formation of the helpline in any way she could. It gave her some purpose. And so the National Hereditary Breast Cancer Helpline began.

I don't particularly remember the first call. It didn't seem much different from the type of calls I had been receiving unofficially for ages. Then the launch by Liz Dawn – Vera Duckworth of *Coronation Street* – brought in an avalanche of further calls, many of which were from people who had been refused referral by their GP. Many GPs were still unaware of the hereditary factors associated with breast cancer, or that the gene could be passed down through the male line. With still so much work to do, I now felt a burgeoning responsibility. I had been asked to set up this service; for sure I had a duty to educate everyone in the sphere of hereditary risk.

And so the busiest year of my life continued at break-neck speed, throwing me first one way then another. Everything worked out smoothly with our move. BT accommodated us with a superb telephone number. Becky continued to grow into a teenager, getting into mischief with her friends, full of fun and happiness. For the first time since we moved to the Peak District, Chris could just go to work and come home without having to mend tractors, as had happened at the farm, or help with the endless duties in a fourteen-hour-a-day shop. I was obviously distracted by the Helpline, but this certainly made far less demands on him. Beryl was adopted into a family, and was happy again. Loneliness must be the cruellest state. The helpline flourished. Gareth and Ros were superb with their support, providing suggestions and solutions over the more difficult helpline requests. I continued to learn about every research study to be sure that all the information would be at my fingertips.

I was invited to attend numerous conferences as a speaker. The first of these had been in Stickney, at the Pilgrim Hospital. As I was introduced, the surgeon tasked with introducing me stated he was really looking forward to this. He said he had often wondered how he would react if asked to perform this operation. Now was his chance to see the effect for himself.

I walked to the front, looking at the sea of faces, grateful for my stage experience which helped me to fight any nerves. I suddenly hit on an idea. I needed to amuse them in the first sentence, so I decisively said, 'Well, I have made a few notes for this, but do you know what I am going to do with them?' I then screwed them up in a ball and threw them over my shoulder. 'This,' I said. It brought a laugh, and from then on I told the story almost as a comedy routine; the cows, the different sizes of prosthetics . . . anything to make it entertaining. They were a great audience.

Gareth fixed up many more of these events. He was involved with a European consortium discussing 'Psycho-social aspects of genetic testing for breast cancer'. I was asked to give the patient's perspective, both my own, and the views and problems encountered through this unique helpline. The first of these meetings was in Germany, in Heidelberg. What a beautiful place. Professor Neva Haites from Aberdeen was the co-ordinator and made a real fuss of me. I enjoyed this experience tremendously.

The media interest continued, with virtually every woman's magazine and newspaper wanting to do a story. An Australian TV programme, *60 Minutes*, had seen the *Decision* documentary, and wanted to reproduce this in Australia; a Japanese company was wanting to film me. It seemed endless. I had really opened a box of knowledge and, hopefully, very quickly, the world would begin to understand it all.

1997: THE GENE PATENT ISSUE

I had prepared the whole cost benefits scheme of funding genetic services, based on genetic test costs of £500 per capita. In the mid-1990s, Myriad Genetics filed a patent application in the USA on BRCA1, the same gene about which my family had contributed valuable research material.

I had already completed many interviews on this subject, rather mesmerized that anyone could patent a human gene. *Horizon* made a TV programme about this. I had challenged the legality of any patent on the discovery of a gene that had used genetic material from willing contributors, in the cause of research and to help others. It all seemed absurd to me. I was probably too candid for my own good, but I was fairly insouciant about what they did in America. It was, I supposed, up to them.

I was nevertheless amazed to receive a call from a lady called Helena, from the Gaia Foundation. Helena had read about my challenge to Myriad's patent, and she wondered if I was aware of an imminent change in European law; a directive to make genes patentable? To begin with, I didn't have the faintest clue what she was talking about and wondered why she was calling me. Then the penny dropped. She spent some time explaining what was actually going on.

Evidently the Genetic Interest Group (GIG) was becoming a strong presence in the European Parliament, persuading MEPs to vote in favour of this proposed directive, which so strongly supported the patenting of genes. I couldn't understand the rationale behind it at all. I heard there was a meeting in London, a patients' meeting, and invited myself along. It was clear my presence wasn't particularly welcome. Nevertheless I battled on. I asked why they were so pro-patenting when clearly this would be a step backwards in many instances.

'Take the breast cancer genes for example,' I insisted. 'This would make genetic testing miles too expensive! At the moment the cost to our NHS is around £500, yet Myriad charges $2,400.'

I explained the implications of all this for patients, and was cut short. The meeting ended fairly quickly.

I was still baffled over this, and vowed to find out more. Helena was extremely helpful. She told me more about the document, and sent it to me. I remember that deep within the second half of the layers of 'bureaucratic speak', appeared this small section:

1. A gene is not patentable.

2. Notwithstanding that, an element isolated from the human body by means of a technical procedure including a gene or partial gene sequence may be patentable.

So, what does one make of that little riddle? Your average lay person is going to assume that the document is stating that genes aren't patentable in any form. They are led to believe the technical procedure is the patentable item, but read it again. And again.

I decided the only real way of finding out whether this meant that a gene *would* be patentable was to ring up the two patent offices, the UK office in Cardiff and the European office, and ask them straight: if this law is passed will it mean that genes are patentable in the context of a genetic test?

The answer was 'yes'.

I now realised what was actually going on; the initial idea to try to wrap it up in a way that was vaguely misleading. In fact, in my later visits to the European Parliament, many MEPs were clearly of this impression. 'It's the technical procedure which will be patentable,' was the regular, inaccurate, response to my concerns.

Once back in the UK, armed with all the knowledge, I contacted all the government ministers and MPs I could find. My first port of call was my long-suffering geneticist, friend and advisor, Gareth Evans, to find out his view. Would this patenting of genes really be helpful or not? The answer was a resounding 'no'. Gareth was appalled. I also contacted the person in the Department of Health whose job it was to take care of such issues. His name was Tony Chapman. The responses were astounding in their lack of 'get up and go'. They ranged from a fairly concerned minister, Joan Ruddock, to the Department of Health, all stating they were keeping their eye on the issue. Oh my goodness, what use was that? The vote was only a matter of weeks away. I even wrote to Tony Blair, but received a fairly noncommittal response, stating he was aware of this. Oh good! How helpful.

The next thing was to alert the media which was not so easy. This was not the subject to stir the imaginations of your average journalist. It was hardly sexy or stimulating news, yet in itself it was enormously important. But eventually the broadsheets started to take it up and pretty soon I was receiving phone calls from all the newspapers, wanting to discuss the issues. Plus, there was a hook for this story: my commitment to genetic tests for breast cancer, my personal story, and my family's contribution to the discovery of this gene.

Before I knew where I was, the *Independent* allotted me an entire page with the headline, 'The Body In Question Is Mine'. The *Sunday Times* wrote extensively on the subject – 'Women's Anger over Cancer Gene Patents' – and so on until the *Guardian* reported, 'Wendy Watson, spearheading the campaign against the gene patent directive'.

Oh my goodness, good grief, blooming heck ... WHAT?!

I had not intended to spearhead anything of the sort. Surely it was up to politicians, the Department of Health, the newspapers, or some other official body to lead this? Not Wendy Watson, sitting in her cottage in the Derbyshire Peak District, running a little helpline and looking after a needy family. Surely it should be someone more 'official' doing this? The idea was totally nuts and, as usual, I got the giggles.

Pretty soon I was contacted by most leading radio programmes to discuss the topic. I was invited to a debate to represent the 'anti-patent' lobby in a debate on the World Service, pitched against Ed Lenz from SmithKlein Beecham in America. Flipping heck. He would have been in briefing meetings for the past six months. I was fresh from making beans on toast for a demanding teenager. Crazy.

To me the whole thing was obvious. Why patent entire genes when this surely would inhibit research? The pharmaceutical line was that without patents there was no incentive to carry out research. My line was that, *with* patents on the entire genes, there was no incentive to continue any research or invest any venture capital in this. If you 'owned' the gene, why not sit there until some university (or similar erudite body) develops a fantastic cure or test using that gene, then proudly stick your hand up in the air and say, 'Aha, that's my gene, I want this amount of licence fee, that amount in royalties', etc.

I discussed all my thoughts, ideas and worries with Gareth Evans, our advisor. He was immediately of the same opinion. He raised this with The British Society of Human Genetics, who then issued a statement. Andrew Read stated that most genes were found as a result of a collaborative approach, and that it was wrong that the person to put the 'last brick in the wall' should be granted the patent. Gareth also wrote a letter that the vast majority of geneticists signed up to, arguing the very points and concerns I had figured out. He stated that, 'The patenting of genes will not foster research; it will kill it.' We argued the point. By all means allow patents on particular medicines using the gene, but not the gene itself. I was coming from an entirely naive angle of fairness, reward for innovation, not for simple financial reward.

Worse was to come. Helena told me that a massive lobby was being orchestrated out in the European Parliament. It was Alastair Kent and his patient groups under the umbrella name of GIG, the outfit I had visited a couple of months before, and its European counter-part EAGS, The European Alliance of Genetic Support Groups. We researched the patient groups who had been approached by GIG to go out to the European Parliament and their instructions.

The programme for the Strasbourg Rally of EAGS patient representatives confirmed their booking into the Holiday Inn. They would be given brochures, posters and T-shirts and could cool down in the hotel swimming pool after the vote. I spoke to Simon Gentry from SmithKline Beecham myself. He, I believe, had the remit to liaise here. Alastair Kent was now kingpin being President of EAGS and Director of GIG. He was also very influential at home as his role was in lobbying for services for patients with rare genetic disorders. He criticized me openly in letters to newspapers, yet I had done nothing wrong. Many others totally agreed with me. The interesting points were GIG's previous vows against patenting genes.

In June 1993, Alastair Kent had written to the Department of Trade and Industry on behalf of GIG to oppose patenting of human genes. He had distinguished the patenting of sequences, which might be acceptable, from that of individual genes, which he opposed:

'Those with most to gain from developments in this field, namely the families affected by genetic disorders, are concerned that their interests will be overlooked in the pressure from others with an interest in extending patent protection for commercial reasons.'

What had changed since then? Now, Alastair was quoted in newspapers in Brussels:

'"The patenting of biotechnology is essential for the application of modern and innovative technology to the prevention and cure of disease," said the organisation's president Alastair Kent. "People suffering from disease urgently need treatments and cures for their conditions. This will only be possible with a secure patent system. Eighty-five per cent of known diseases have no effective treatment, let alone cure."'

I had been in touch with a company called Affymatrix in Santa Barbara, California. They had developed a gene chip which could read up to 50 genes at once, which would speed results. They told me the problem they had in the USA was that, due to patent protection, they could not get this off the ground as so many of the genes for different diseases were 'owned' by different companies. This made the concept unworkable. Some would allow them a licence; others either wouldn't or made it prohibitively expensive. This was exactly the point we were making. The breast cancer genes were precisely a demonstration of what could happen to the costs of testing with single genes. The Affymatrix innovation was a casualty of wide gene patents.

So what to do now? I decided to take one step at a time. I wrote to High Court Patent Law judge Hugh Laddie, asking his advice.

'If this law was to be passed,' I asked, 'would Myriad Genetics be able to extend their patent here and would there be anything I could do about this?'

The very amenable judge rang me one morning, very early. He confirmed that certainly, if Myriad's patent were granted here, then we would have to co-operate. He said there was a compulsory licence law which might help and also put me in touch with a very friendly barrister. Hugh Laddie understood my concerns: it was not so much that Myriad would not allow testing, more that it would become way too expensive for the NHS to cover, thus would effectively cost lives. This was my contention.

The next thing I needed to do was to fly out to the European Parliament to lobby MEPs myself, prior to the vote. If Alastair Kent from GIG could do it, so could Wendy Watson from the Hereditary Breast Cancer

Helpline. I must admit I was quite wary, though. At this stage I had no idea how much had been invested in this pro-patent lobby, just that it must be a significant figure. How I was placed to fight against this 'might', I had no idea. All I could do was talk from the heart, from my own common sense and research findings. I would try to plead the cause for all those who might not get a gene test for breast cancer, despite having a strong family history, and speak on behalf of those who might be denied a test just because the cost would become too great. How much would that cost in real terms? How many lives? Whenever I got really nervous, wondering whether I should chicken out, those thoughts always pulled me back on track. So many parties and members of the public were now relying on me. I was receiving faxes constantly, saying how important my message was in all of this and how I was crucial to the whole 'anti-patent' lobby.

Matt Youdale, our local BBC Health Correspondent, came with me on one of these trips, as did Gareth. Although this was one of the most newsworthy things that had ever happened to me, most people just couldn't get it. It was too much, having to ponder over EU directives, genes and patents. I didn't really want to bore people, yet it had taken over my life at that moment.

During the week of the vote I was back and forth to Brussels and Strasbourg. I was interviewed three times on the *Today Programme* that week. On one occasion John Humphrys set Alastair Kent and me against each other. Alastair was refusing to give a straight answer over the patenting issue, yet he was involved with this lobby urging MEPs to vote for this directive.

In June 1997, a pamphlet entitled *Patents for Life* was

distributed amongst MEPs with the EAGS logo and their heading European Alliance of Genetic Support Groups, stating:

'European Alliance of Genetic Support Groups has been actively involved in the debate on the proposed directive on the patenting of biological inventions. For patients with genetic disorders this proposal is a real question of life or death – in order to have any hope of a cure, longer life or improved heath [*sic*] patients need this Directive.'

In other words, don't listen to such as me, vote for genes to be patentable.

By this time, all the broadsheet newspapers had referred to me as the campaign leader. Many interested groups against the directive and gene patenting contacted me, sending me all the evidence they had amassed, and even more astonishingly asking me what the next step forward should be! I had no idea of course, I was making this up as I went along. I had satisfied myself that despite all the verbose language attempting to send ambiguous, confusing messages about clarification and harmonisation, a simple phone call to the Patent Office confirmed that, yes, with this directive, genes would become legally patentable.

I was inundated with faxes, photocopies and all manner of materials in addition to my own research. I was sent copies of letters Alastair Kent had sent to others over a four-year period, originally opposing broad gene patenting. Had he changed his position over this time? In 1993 he was picked up on the very point that a gene, either 'inside or outside the body', should not be patentable. Now alternative arguments were being put forward. Eloquent but incomprehensible wording could easily cast doubt as to what was what, but if people needed to know exactly, why not do as I did and ask the experts? Did EAG and GIG have different attitudes and if so, which side of the gene argument did Alastair Kent support? I could not work out where he stood on the *Patents for Life* leaflet issued for the European Alliance of Genetic Support groups he was president of. If I could ascertain that the directive meant genes would be patentable, why couldn't he? And also, why did lobbyists fly out patients in wheelchairs to sit outside the European Parliament and promote 'patents for life' if it was against broad gene patents?

George Monbiot wrote an article for a newspaper, entitled 'Beware the Wheelchairs' stating this was the hardest essay he could ever write. He concluded his article:

'Next week, disabled people, funded by corporations, will be tugging once more upon the heartstrings of our MEPs as they make the final decision about whether to allow a handful of companies to claim us as their own. It's the last chance they'll have to resist these monstrous demands and show that emotional blackmail doesn't pay.'

I have to leave the reader to decide. Various reports on the internet claim multi-million pound investments into this patient lobby. I have no proof of that, just the evidence of the conflicting and confusing copious propaganda.

I amassed an enormous amount of material, faxes and suchlike from the GIG establishment. Other patient groups sent them on to me. I still have boxes of all of this material and copies of everything at my local solicitor's office – I was taking no chances. Politically, the debate really hotted up. I received *Hansard* which gives the exact transcript of everything said in Parliament. The Royal Society issued a statement opposing the patenting of genetic material, stating that commercial pressures in this direction pose a grave threat to scientific research and a hindrance to its ultimate medical applications. It was clear that the current government was terrified of losing our pharmaceutical industry via their threats if this directive was not passed. I doubted this. Empty threats in my estimation, but enough to scare our politicians.

It was also during this time that the helpline became busier. All the publicity I was creating about the gene patent stimulated interest in the inherited factors of breast cancer. I felt as if my life had just gone totally silly. How could I, the person who loved practical jokes, singing, and amateur theatre have become embroiled in this? Talk about from the sublime to the totally and utterly ridiculous!

Of course, try as I might, I could not have altered the minds of the MEPs who genuinely believed that what these patients were lobbying for – patent protection for the pharmaceutical industry on genes – was the general feeling. Lots of people were supportive, but there was only one of me.

So, the vote was approved which was a triumph for GIG and the SKB lobby. I hoped I had had some effect as it did not score such a great majority as was hoped.

All was not lost though. I had spent months researching patent law and had already challenged the American Myriad patent; I was ready for the European onslaught. I had raised awareness of this all over Europe. I expect I was viewed as some cranky female who had not only had her breasts chopped off but was now charging round Europe like a maniac. The UK patent office, in particular an extremely helpful man called Derek, used to answer my calls every day, in my bid to learn everything I could about patent law.

Many civil servants and politicians thought we could just ignore any patent application on the genes. They assumed that the Department of Health would be exempt from these laws. I knew differently. I had read up on the TRIPS (Trade Related Intellectual Property) agreement, which was part of the World Trade Organization. I knew with great certainty that this was a naive hope, that it just wouldn't happen. Within world trade agreements, the imagined immunity of the Department of Health in the UK would easily be swept aside. We would all be severely affected.

I was now a woman on a mission!

As I had predicted, Myriad filed their patent application in the whole of Europe. Denmark took the case on, challenging the validity of some of the sequencing; I merely challenged the patent on the grounds of it contravening the essence of patent law itself:

'Part 4. Must not be contrary to public morality.'

Yes, it clearly would be. Straightforward diagnostic tests would become too expensive for the NHS. Rationing would be further introduced leading to lives being lost. As simple as that. By this time, risk-reducing surgery was being reported regularly, with several small studies published demonstrating overwhelming evidence that the procedure worked. It reduced breast cancer incidences by over 90 per cent. Therefore it saved lives.

As it happened, Myriad's patent application in Europe was defeated, saving us all millions of pounds.

We are currently saving around £8,000,000 per year on patent costs, the difference between our own laboratory costs and Myriad's highly inflated $3,000. Since figures have been collated by the CMGS (Clinical Molecular Genetic Society) we have now in the UK performed 36,273 mutation screens and 9,627 predictive tests, at a net saving of £55,780,946 since data began! Big numbers to take in. I'm just glad and proud I had the guts to do my small bit in all of this.

In fact, quite remarkably, my fight has become a discussion module in the Council on Science and Technology at Princeton University, under Professor Richard Pierre Claude – 'The case of Wendy Watson versus Myriad Genetics'. I'm sure if they actually met me they would marvel that a university course (especially somewhere as august as Princeton) could be modelled on such a hapless female. To be honest, I giggle every time I think of it.

Alastair Kent holds a lofty position on the Government's Human Genetic Commission, and is still chair of the Genetic Interest Group, now renamed the Genetic Alliance UK.

Sisters Andrea and Rhonda had their operations in 1997. There was more media attention. The show called *60 Minutes* in Australia decided to focus on Andrea and Rhonda, rather than just re-enacting our family's story. The lovely producer flew over for several weeks and filmed Andrea and Rhonda in exactly the style of *The Decision*. I kept in close contact with the girls. They were regular visitors and obviously had many questions as the time for their operations grew closer. We grew very fond of each other. I felt a personal responsibility towards them. True, they had made their own decisions, but I had facilitated these objectives. I needn't have worried, however; they both sailed through the surgery under the genius work of Andrew Baildam, now Chair of the British Association of Surgeons, BASO.

Andrea chose to have the same procedure as I had done – a total mastectomy. Rhonda chose a more cosmetic approach. She had the breast tissue removed, but kept her own nipples, and opted for immediate reconstruction using implants. Andrea was already married and had two small children; Rhonda was single. It is, of course, important for everyone to feel comfortable with whatever choice they make regarding surgery or non-surgery, reconstruction or no reconstruction. Clearly though, for anyone as yet unmarried, the issue is easier to deal with if a reasonable cosmetic result can be achieved. We remained firm friends throughout and now both girls have survived way past the ages reached by their mum and grandma.

Several years later I received the following letter from Andrea:

Dear Wendy

I have just been reading the experiences of others with family histories of breast cancer on your website. It took me right back to when you were helping me through this situation. It was 13 years ago, when I saw a documentary about you on TV. I wrote a letter explaining that my mother had died at 31 of breast cancer and my grandmother had been just 26. I wasn't really expecting that you would do anything to help me but it was a great relief to be telling someone who would understand how frightening it is to think that you will be next. I was 25 at the time and my children were two and one. I was so scared that they would have to grow up without me. You called me the very next day. You talked me through everything. Over the next few months I was constantly on the phone to you and you were always so patient and helpful. You went through the whole process with me from understanding my risks to the bilateral mastectomy. Back then it was difficult to get the medical profession to even consider removing healthy breast tissue. You helped me fight the local NHS trust to get the funding I needed for my treatment. I think the fact that women are no longer looked at as if they are crazy for even thinking about preventative mastectomies has a lot to do with the work you have done and the positive way in which you have handled your own situation. You were one of the first people to visit me in the hospital and I was so pleased to see you.

My life has gone on and I'm pleased to say I have never looked back. I have not regretted for one moment the decision I made. Reading the comments of others has reminded me how vital it was to have someone to talk to. Someone who understood and who would do anything she could to help. I'm so glad that you are still there for all those women who need you. You should be so proud of the work that you and Becky do. You have changed so many lives and probably saved many lives. My children are 15 and 13 now and they have not had to watch their mother suffer breast cancer as I did growing up. So, thank you, Wendy. I owe you so much.

Keep up the good work.

Love, Andrea

I find it extraordinarily difficult to read that without a tear or a lump in my throat.

RUNNING THE HELPLINE

From 1998 life took a calmer turn for several years. I continued to run the helpline with the assistance of the Small Government Section 64 grant. I carried on running Peak Performance and producing shows at Buxton. I still belonged to several operatic and drama groups and still adored being on stage. The excitement of standing in the wings, the dread of what might go wrong and how you would get out of it is completely addictive. Of course, I was out rehearsing most nights, trying to grab every moment and loving it all so much. Peak Performance had now become a well-respected group of amateur and professional actors, singers and musicians. Many of the children who started with us in musicals such as *Oliver* have now gone on to make it to the big time. In particular, cute little Emma Hopkinson, the tiniest thing ever, stole everyone's heart in the title role of *Oliver* with her big voice that just knocked you back. Emma went on to win the lead in a professional production of *Annie*, with Sue Pollard, touring Britain. Michael, our other Oliver, started many ventures and theatre companies himself. He gained a place at a top theatre school. Tom, our hero in *South Pacific*, recently featured in the fantastic 25-year celebration of *Les Miserables* at the O2. He was the opening soloist. It is not without some pride that I hope we at least gave some impetus, encouragement and experience to these youngsters.

We were asked to write a show in 1999 to celebrate the centenary of Buxton Opera House. I called it simply *Journey Through 100 Years of Song* – excerpts from shows, comedy song-and-dance routines, all coloured through a massive costume and lighting plot. This too went down a storm.

Each year, the company put on shows to raise awareness of hereditary breast cancer. I would like to say we raised money for the helpline, but usually the costs exceeded the revenue. It was a brilliant exercise in publicity though. As I was dancing around the stage, taking many leading roles, I hoped I could inspire others with a positive example. The newspapers loved it. The idea was to raise awareness, but any profits were to be donated to the helpline and the cause. Sadly, even with packed houses profit is hard to make, but the profits from *Annie* led us to produce our first information leaflets for the public.

Back at home, Beryl became quite poorly, and carers would look after her in the evenings. In the daytimes everything was fine. I was there manning the helpline, and all Beryl asked was my love and company, and to be hugged and cuddled regularly; this was so easy to give. Her only concern, which I had to reassure her about constantly, was that I would not leave her or put her in a home. Poor Beryl. I promised I would never ever do that. She would then relax and smile with tears in her eyes. I can say no more on this, but her death in 1998 was so sad. At least she stayed at home.

In 1998, having spoken at the European consortium on hereditary breast cancer in Heidelberg, I was asked to continue this same theme throughout Europe. This was chiefly to give the patient perspective, but now, in addition, to provide intelligence from the Helpline data. I travelled to Marseilles Frankfurt, Barcelona and Paris.

After a year or so, I found that answering the helpline was second nature. I soon began to understand how to listen to people's concerns, and to empathizes without offering an opinion or being drawn into debate, but trying to present a balanced view while keeping a positive note. Pretty soon I had received professional endorsements from most leading geneticists. Professor Sandy Raeburn from Nottingham regularly asked me to teach his student group. We had become firm friends and he showed his support by his frequent contact and referral of his patients to my service.

I had thousands of callers, some easily satisfied with the more simple explanation of where to be referred next. Many, though, became like a personal friend for as long as they needed me. Reading their letters and cards was always extremely warming and thrilling. To think that just talking with someone could have, as Baroness Cumberlege said, 'a profound effect' on them, was moving for me.

Initially, I had set up the helpline as a Monday to Friday 9 a.m.– 5 p.m. service, but eventually always answered the phone whenever I was at home in the evening and at night. I had had a small increase in the grant to enable me to employ an assistant. Neither of us received much in the way of payment. I started, though, to have a couple of hours off in the afternoons. The advent of the BT 'CallDivert' service, allowing the phone to be diverted anywhere – even to my mobile – led to the line actually being answered 24 hours a day, just because it was possible. At first, the out-of-hours demand was not that great, but soon it became apparent that evenings and weekends were really the only times many of the callers were able to get a few minutes to themselves in privacy, as they couldn't possibly call in work hours. It was the difficulty of discussing the issue with work colleagues or friends that was a driving force in the helpline being needed so much. I just sort of slipped into the 24-hour mode, and apparently still remain one of the only helpline services open night and day.

Financially, as long as I could manage to pay the bills, I was happy with the grant. I worked from home and had enough money to pay a small wage to Becky to man the phones in the afternoons. The work was immensely rewarding and money has never been a driving force for me. Yes, we all need enough to live, and so did I. It was paramount that this would be possible, but I don't think I have ever been greedy in this respect. I have continued to live my life fully around the helpline.

In the late 1990s, I received a call from a young girl from Aberdeen called Maria. Her story was more tragic than most. Her mother had died from breast cancer when she was very young, and her aunt followed very quickly. Another of Maria's aunts soon contracted the disease but so far has survived it. Maria had been very close to this aunt through her upbringing. She initially played a significant part in Maria's life, being there for her through her wedding to John, whom Maria describes as her wonderful rock. She also helped through the birth of Maria's first two children, until family upsets occurred. Then everything changed; Maria herself decided to undergo testing; the family had donated 'bloods' for research purposes.

Due to a family feud, which had nothing to do with the gene testing issue, her aunt removed permission to use the sample as a comparative. She said she 'wouldn't hand her DNA over on a plate'. To this day Maria has no idea why this rift should have had such a devastating effect on the 10 millilitres of blood required for a genetic test. Maria was desperate to undergo this test. As she saw it, it would prove whether or not she may have inherited the faulty breast cancer gene running in her family. This would open the door for further options. The aunt had not only removed her permission for her blood sample to be used, but also refused to speak about this with Maria, who was understandably devastated.

During these years of testing, Maria was trying desperately for a family. She had six miscarriages before she was diagnosed with anticardiolipin – a blood clotting disease. This was treated successfully, allowing Maria to carry three beautiful children to full term. There were concerns, though, of undergoing any elective operations without confirmation of the presence of a gene fault – especially given the extra health risk of any surgery at all with anticardiolipin.

We spoke many times on the phone and eventually I felt I should drive over and meet her. The whole family seemed to be against Maria, for reasons she neither knew of, nor could even imagine. Her loyal husband remained staunchly supportive throughout. Maria's three small children kept her focused on her goal: to see them grow up and to put the shadow of breast cancer firmly behind her.

We arranged to meet one freezing cold Sunday in Penrith. We walked around the cold, rainy and depressingly empty town centre until we found a cheerful pub which served meals. For the next three hours we talked non-stop with Maria spilling out her story. She told me of the heartbreak at losing her mum, and now her mum's sister denying her help. The family would not speak of this, other than blaming her for causing upsets. She wanted her children to be involved with their grandparents, but sadly this was not to be.

Maria wanted to know about my story, and how I had had to make choices before any genetic tests were available. Given the high incidence of very young breast cancers in Maria's family, there was possibly only one route left, namely to make a decision without a test. For many, this is the only option, but Maria had also to face the disapproval, lack of support and, indeed, ostracism from her family, in addition to possible medical complications.

For months she would write to me, or we would phone and she was to tell me later that I was all she had. I found that unutterably sad, and felt devastated for her. It's one thing to have to make these choices, but quite another to have your family turn their back on you in the process. Maria and I kept in touch regularly through those next few months. I lived those months with her in my head, every conversation making me wish I could do something more to help. I was so mindful to be careful not to influence her in any way, but making a decision without a test result was the stark choice for her.

She wrote to me after her decision to go ahead with surgery, telling me of its success, and saying how much she had valued my support as I was all she had during that time.

Over the next few years, I was to receive many calls from Scotland. One girl, Lorraine, had suffered so many traumas one way or another, it seemed unbearable. I was once again totally saddened to hear of the lack of support from her family – something which, thankfully, had never been an issue for me.

Lorraine had been given the helpline number by one of the larger cancer charities, either Macmillan or Breast Cancer Care, as they had little expertise in the genetic risk area. From the outset, I realised that Lorraine was having an awful time. Her parents had divorced when she was a baby, and she had had no contact with her father. Her sister got in touch with Lorraine when she was in her early thirties to tell her that, in addition to their grandparents' cancers on their father's side, their father's sister – their aunt – had also now developed breast cancer. The aunt had undergone a genetic test and had been diagnosed as carrying the faulty BRCA2 gene. The hospital which had carried out the genetic test had also informed other relatives to see if they wished to be tested themselves. Lorraine took the decision to undergo testing and was now waiting to see if she too carried the fault.

Initially, the genetics team and Lorraine decided she should have a mammogram to put her mind at rest while she researched all her options. This was to prove one of the most difficult days in this girl's life. Here is the distraught and heart-rending email I received from her:

Hi Wendy,

How are you? I thought I would let you know that I had a mammogram carried out yesterday which was probably one of the worst experiences ever. The actual test itself was fine and the nurse performing the test was amazing, however the breast GP was a nightmare.

When I arrived at the hospital I was led into a room and was then met with the consultant/radiographer. After reading through my notes he advised that I wouldn't be getting the mammogram as he didn't think I had BRCA2. He based this conclusion on the fact that he has been a doctor for over 20 years and he has only come across a few people with the gene. The things he said to me were astonishing, such as after asking the history in the family he asked if I could see a pattern with the amount of women in the family with breast cancer. When I told him no he said, 'See, it's mostly women that are getting it so you probably won't have it as it shouldn't be passed through your dad.' When I told him my grandfather and his four brothers all died of cancer and his sisters had died also he still tried to tell me I was wrong and said my dad's aunts and uncles are irrelevant as they were not my direct gene link. I informed him my dad's sister has breast cancer and his other two sisters have tested positive for the gene, he said he knew but again they were women. He asked me a few times if there was cancer in my mum's side of the family. When I told him "no" he said that I should stop worrying then. He also said that he is fifty-something per cent sure I won't have it.

Wendy, what was very disturbing was when he was asking me things about the gene and when I said I was concerned he looked at the nurse and continued to do a silly laugh and raise his eyes and shrug his shoulders making me feel I had absolutely no right whatsoever to be there. When he read that I wanted to discuss preventive surgery if the result was positive he was annoyed as he said, 'Women should stop rushing into having their breasts removed as it doesn't solve the problem.' He asked me, 'Do you know how many people will get cancer in their lifetime?' and I said probably about one in eight, as I wasn't sure. Again he laughed and said, 'No, one in four, so what does that mean? Should we go about removing people's vital organs just in case they get cancer?' He also said he noticed I will get a reduction if results are negative and said that wasn't the answer to giving me peace of mind as often there will be more lumps and can look awful. When I told him when I examine myself I can feel lumps he said I couldn't and again I said I could. He said, 'No dear, you feel glands.' But how am I supposed to know? I'm not a breast expert . . . He said I probably won't even get a reduction if this is negative as my GP also has to refer me and I would need to make sure I was prepared mentally for it. In the end he said he will ask for a mammogram from the X-ray dept and if they say no he will call my genetics counsellor and ask why on earth I was sent for one. If I write down a list of the family history of who has died he may consider doing it at a later date. Thankfully they said they would do it a few hours later and when I returned for the results I was first led back into that room. When he came he led me out to the corridor where there were two patients and three nurses and discussed my results. Even then he said he will probably see me again as this will come back negative and I will just be referred for screenings every two/three years.

Wendy, it has been very hard writing this email as that man really upset me. When he left the room I thought I will never return for more results or tests again and perhaps he was correct. Maybe I am overreacting by wanting to find out? I still don't know what to do now as I feel I am trying

*to deal with my close relatives fighting cancer and knowing
I could carry the gene. I honestly cannot continue to be
made to feel like that as I always thought these apparently
professional people were supposed to help you, not make you
worse. If he doesn't understand genetics he shouldn't
discuss it or push his silly opinions on very vulnerable,
obviously worried women and men. I certainly shouldn't
leave these appointments in tears or being sick and wondering if it's worth the hassle.*
Love, Lorraine xx

I advised Lorraine to go back to the genetic service
and book yet another appointment with her counsellor, whom I spoke to myself. I really felt the attitude of
this medic was not only inappropriate, but he had also
got his facts wrong. Of course, the gene can be passed
down through the male line, and I was very concerned
that a medical person should try to convince someone
otherwise.

Several people in Scotland seemed to have very difficult problems all at the same time. I tried to put them
all in touch with one another, and it soon became apparent that for everyone to meet would be the best way
forward. We were kindly donated a venue for a couple
of days in the Highlands – which happened to be a
castle! Everyone was tremendously excited by this;
Maria's children were totally enchanted by the prospect of playing fairy princesses in the turrets.

The plan was to bring a joint feast for the first evening.
I was the last to arrive, having travelled for about seven
hours. What a welcome I received! Maria opened the
castle door and I was blown away by her new look.
Gone was the pitiful girl I had met on that dreary day
in Penrith; in her place stood a bubbly, happy and

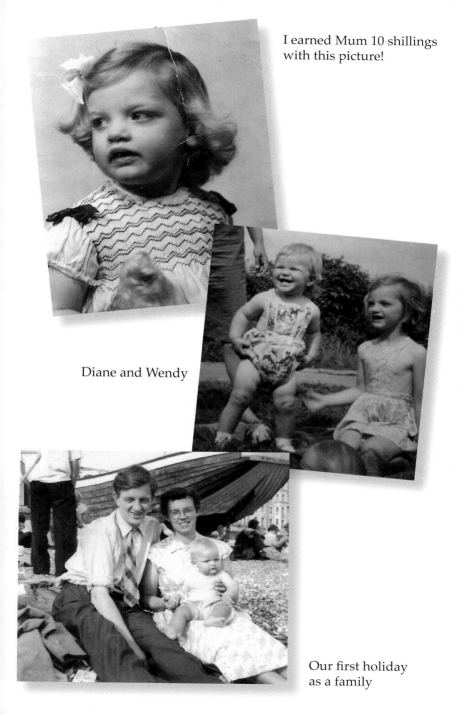

I earned Mum 10 shillings with this picture!

Diane and Wendy

Our first holiday as a family

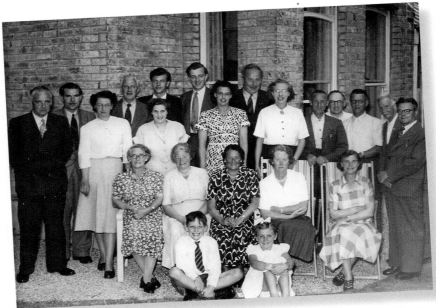

Mum and Dad's engagement

Becky as an innocent toddler? Hmmm . . .

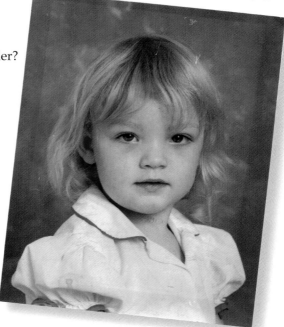

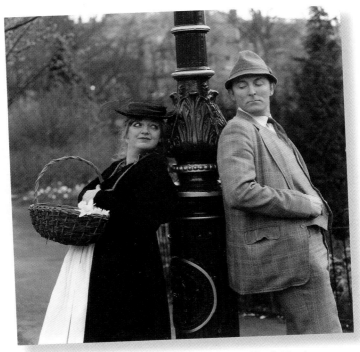

Peak Performance's first show, *My Fair Lady* at Buxton Opera House, 1996. Gareth and Wendy playing the leading roles

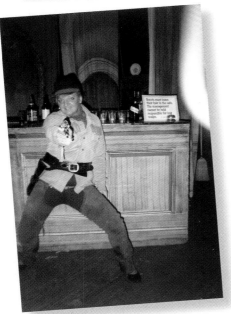

Having fun playing the eponymous role in *Calamity Jane*. Life definitely begins at 40!

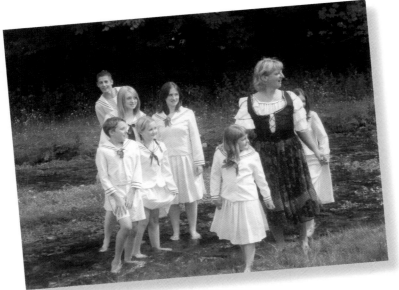

Wendy as Maria in *The Sound of Music*, Buxton Opera House, 2006. Peak Performance 10 years on and still going strong

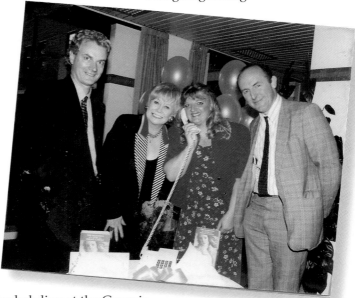

Launch of the helpline at the Genesis Appeal Centre with patron Liz Dawn

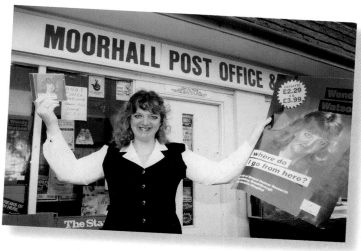

The launch of the fundraising single *Where do I Go from Here?* Hereditary Breast Cancer Awareness week, 1996

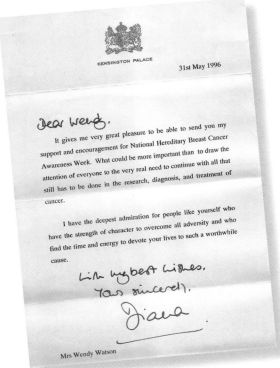

Princess Diana's wonderful support letter

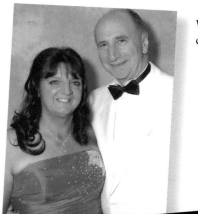

Wendy and husband Chris at the charity ball at Chatsworth House, 2010

Rhonda and Andrea celebrate reaching 40 with surgeon Andrew Baildam, Charity Ball, Chatsworth

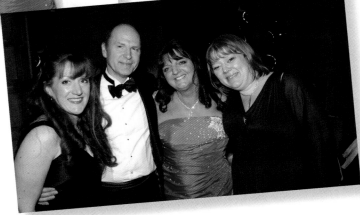

Skydivers at Langar Airfield, all wearing their nominated PCT t-shirts in aid of the helpline

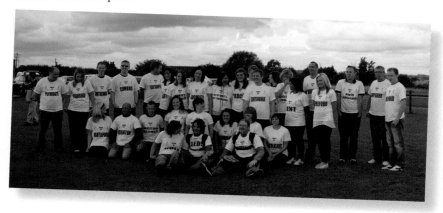

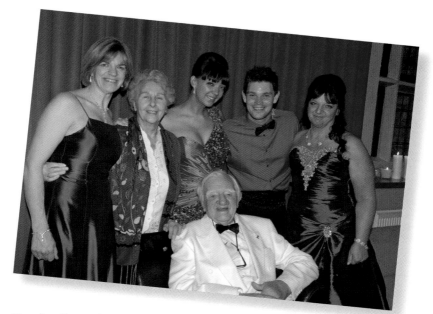

Our family at the Thornbridge Hall Charity Ball

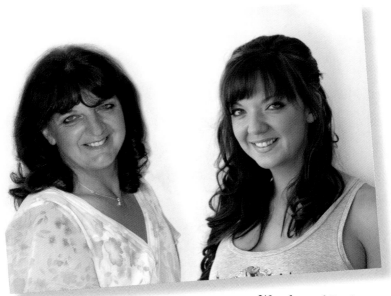

Wendy and Becky now

Rt. Hon. ANDY BURNHAM MP
Labour Member of Parliament for Leigh

HOUSE OF COMMONS
LONDON SW1A 0AA

10 MARKET STREET
LEIGH WN7 1DS

Tel: 01942 682353

Ms Wendy Watson
Hereditary Breast Cancer Helpline
St Anne's Cottage
Over Haddon
Derby
DE45 1JE

Our ref AB/cp
14 March 2011

Dear Wendy

It was lovely to meet you earlier in the year and be able to say to you face to face how important I believe the National Hereditary Breast Cancer Helpline to be.

Once again I must offer my apologies as I am not to be able to be with you at your wonderful Gala Ball this year and I hope that it is another really fabulous occasion for the Helpline.

I am thoroughly in admiration of you and your small team as you strive to bring this hugely important matter to public, medical and research prominence.

The knowledge we have now of the genetic influence on breast cancer is highly significant and is, indeed, saving the lives of women of all ages by empowering them to understand their risk factors and take the decisions that are right for each one of them. Your work to support women and their families is tremendous and long may you continue.

I was delighted to hear that you have won the TESCO Mum of the Year, well done, indeed.

I am glad to be able to let you know that my wife, Marie-France, is recovering well from her own surgery and we both thank you for the support you have provided for us and trail-blazing work that you have done to make such treatment possible.

Please pass on my very best wishes to all the people involved with this evening's ball and to all your workers and supporters. I would like to offer a prize for any fundraising you are undertaking (my office will be in touch to arrange this).

Yours sincerely

ANDY BURNHAM

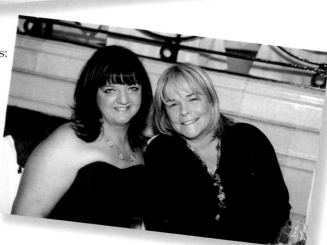

Tesco Mum of the Year Awards: such an emotional and proud moment glowing mum. The memory of what I saw next has made me laugh on so many occasions since.

We climbed the stairs in the north turret to the first floor dining hall. The dining table was about 30 feet long, and was laden with food, looking like a scene from Henry VIII's court. The dining chairs engulfed each child with about a three-foot gap between them. The enormous welcoming log fire crackled in an inglenook fireplace that was the same size as most people's living rooms. Large comfortable sofas and armchairs were arranged in cosy groupings, and one wall lined with a library of books seemingly from the sixteenth century completed the scene. You can imagine the atmosphere. Most people there could never in their wildest dreams imagine a holiday in these surroundings.

The evening was one of sheer jollity, with our several bottles of cheap wine totally out of keeping with the opulence of our cut-glass wine glasses. The children were dashing around from turret to turret, exploring every nook and cranny. They dodged from the quaint little chapel room, complete with pews and an altar, to the eerie dungeons. The extensive attic rooms were converted to sleeping areas, where they all slept together.

After around four hours of laughter, someone said, 'Gosh, I had almost forgotten why we are here.' But of course we were actually doing what we were there to do. To present a life that can be normal despite this ghastly gene and to normalise the situation. The whole weekend worked like a dream. Maria was the life and soul of the party; her husband thanked me and said, 'You gave me back the girl I married.' I had to dash off quickly then as I cry so easily at happy endings.

Lorraine eventually went on to undergo both the removal of her ovaries and a double mastectomy. She sailed through the ovarian operation, but unfortunately had complications with the breast surgery. She experienced very severe problems, which resulted in necrosis of some of the breast tissue.

I have recently been in touch with Lorraine, who had practically given up all hope of looking reasonable. The surgeon, Mr Baildam, agreed to see her if she could get funding from Scotland. After helping Lorraine with many protracted and arduous fights, her health authority has finally conceded that the treatment she received was appalling, and have agreed to her having further surgery in Manchester.

I have truly made so many friends, and their gratitude, which has been overwhelming, was, and is, totally unnecessary: I felt it was so easy for me to help, and it has all been my pleasure. If I won the lottery I would continue exactly as I am now. I really, really love my job, and the brilliant people I have met.

NEW WORLDS TO CONQUER

Dad and Olive wanted a trip to California. They needed us to travel with them, and had loads of plans to circumnavigate the entire state with Chris and me at the wheel. That was fine, not a problem, but I had to face my fear of flying again. I weighed up the risk of flying against the guilt if I wouldn't go – not to mention my genuine desire to see Las Vegas, Disneyland, Universal Studios, Palm Springs and the Grand Canyon for myself. In the end, I agreed to the trip.

No sooner was it all booked, than the Twin Towers horror story unfurled. I felt, as we all did, a tremendous sadness for the families, their devastation, and the terrors of those trapped in the towers and forced to jump to their deaths. I also scarcely dared to think of my prospective flight, booked for 20 October.

Of course, I knew that the airports would be on the highest alerts possible. Just before we were due to leave England for this trip, I received a phone call from Professor James Coyne of the University of Pennsylvania, Philadelphia. I had met James when I was speaking at a psycho-social conference in Marseilles. We had become great friends and he was tremendously interested in setting up a similar helpline service in the USA, and had been keen to try to get me over there. I told him I would be in California until around 10 November, if that was any use. He said he would contact me.

Somehow or other, I mustered up enough courage (and Valium!) to get me to Manchester Airport to fly the two legs of the journey to Las Vegas.

Once on board, I settled myself into my usual superstitious rituals, fulfilling my personal responsibilities for keeping this lump of metal airborne. Somehow, though, being on board a craft as large as this, with cameras to see the view from all angles, was an enormous comfort. We were in an upgrade because Olive, who used to be an airhostess back in the stone age, as she put it, had written to the British Midland boss. He remembered her and kindly upgraded us. This was a different kettle of fish entirely. No need for Valium at all. The champagne to welcome you on board helped enormously.

Of course, after landing at Chicago, we had to repeat the whole experience again with boarding and security, but I made it. In fact, so strong was my willpower over the next plane, it hadn't got a chance of falling out of the sky!

The entire Californian experience was totally unexpected to me. The vastness of the deserts was incredible. I loved Palm Springs and Disneyland. And Universal Studios with the ET bike ride – flying over New York at night with ET sat in my basket was totally magical. But, although I loved it all, I concluded that America was not a country I wanted to live in.

Towards the end of the holiday I received a call saying, 'Professor James Coyne would like you to spend several days in Philadelphia, giving lectures and talks to various people he has got together at the University of Pennsylvania.' The timing of this was lousy: from 14-20 November. I would get back home for a few days only, then have to do it all again. All those aeroplanes!

Eventually Barbara, James's long-suffering PA, came up with a brilliant idea. She invited us to stay at her home in Maryland over the Thanksgiving period, to save us trekking back to England. I had an even better idea. Why not use the four or five days to drive across America and save two air flights? Well, of course, all of these 'know-alls' thought that was a silly idea. Far too far to drive, didn't I realise it was nearly 3,000 miles? I supposed I did, but I was just looking for an 'easy' option for me to take. However, everyone else just dismissed the idea as ludicrous so, in the end, I acquiesced.

We parted from Dad and Olive in Chicago, leaving them to fly back to England without us, and went on to Washington DC, where Barbara met us from the plane. She took us back to her home, which was your typical large family home with a huge basement play area. The family made us really welcome.

Thanksgiving was the reason our visit to the university could not have been directly tagged on to the end of our holiday. And what a total privilege it turned out to be for us, to be part of a real American family celebrating this occasion. I learnt to make a pumpkin pie, and the traditional apple pie, which was much better than ours. We had great fun together. The family took us to the Air and Space Museum, where there is a kind of Perspex tube affair containing a tiny piece of moon rock that you can poke your finger into and touch a piece of the moon. Quirky, gimmicky and great fun.

This brief interlude was quickly followed by the hectic talks schedule that had been arranged for me. They certainly wanted to ensure my time was well spent. Ten lectures per day for three solid days are quite a lot, I reckon! The doctors, consultants, professors and nurses all expressed astonishment at the train of events and circumstances I had to tackle. Events and obstacles which just had to be pushed aside or knocked over in order to get to the people who *can* effect change.

The challenge, as always, was to get those people to listen to the story. You need to be engaging from the outset. I got through the 30 or so talks and lectures though, and made several great contacts. Many people wanted me to stay in the USA and set up a similar service there, but that was not for me. I hadn't realised how much I loved England, even with its ghastly weather. I also had responsibilities back home where Becky, and one of Gareth's genetic counsellors, Rachel Belk, were manning the helpline for me. That was not a sustainable arrangement.

The following year or two carried on in much the same vein, except for a chance request from Jonathan Rowlands. Jonathan lived only a mile or two away from me and knew of the singing and performing I enjoyed so much. Jonathan owned the rights to the Captain Beaky collection of songs, which were very popular, and had interested the National Youth Ballet in performing them at Sadler's Wells. He asked me if I would sing one of the six songs chosen for this performance. Joanna Lumley was also performing. Would I be interested? Would I? You bet I would!

We recorded the song locally and the track was sent to a London studio for mastering. As the date for the performance grew closer, I could scarcely believe that I would be a soloist in this world-famous venue. That event was more than thrilling.

We had the best evening, and the children who were dancing to 'Fred and Marguerite' (about two sparrows!), the song I had recorded, were adorable. They loved the song, and the standard of the choreography and dancing was incredible. Joanna Lumley was wonderful, so friendly. As if this wasn't enough, the following year the same set was performed at the London Palladium. Once again I marvelled at how, totally out of the blue, I should be a soloist in a venue such as this. Suffice it to say, it was one of life's greatest experiences.

What was most thrilling of all was that this show had nothing to do with fundraising, publicity, and breast cancer awareness. No. I had been asked solely on my singing ability and suitability for that particular song. That, to me, was the biggest compliment. Jim Parker, the well-known composer, was hugely complimentary. He thanked me for my wonderful interpretation of the song and said I had a beautiful voice.

Of course, audiences had come to see these first-rate child ballet-dancers performing, not to listen to the singers, but nevertheless I was thrilled to pieces. Seriously, how many people would have the chance to be a soloist in two top London theatres? Never in my wildest dreams could I have imagined it for myself. Dad and Olive came along too, both so proud – Dad of his daughter, and Olive for encouraging my singing in the first place. Jonathan took us all out for a late meal after the show. We were all high on the success, and relived the evening over and over again. This was a far cry from the local operatic societies I performed wih most evenings, although by now Peak Performance had gathered the status of a professionally run local theatre group. Our shows at Buxton Opera House sold extremely well every year.

I learned to play bridge and became totally and utterly addicted to the game. In fact, I almost joined in with the diehards' scorn when anyone had the temerity to call it a 'game'. It was during the early part of this learning process that I received a call to chair a session at a debate in the Church Rooms, Westminster. The debate was, of course, on genetic testing for breast cancer. It was to be held on a Tuesday night, which unfortunately clashed with my bridge course, but they were most conciliatory and agreed to hold my session in the morning.

My bridge partner asked me who had organized the debate. I told him it was The Royal Society. The Royal Society of what, he enquired; GPs, nurses, physicians maybe? I had no idea. All I caught was the name, Royal Society. Eventually I discovered that this organization was known simply as 'The Royal Society'. When I relayed this to my bridge partner he spluttered, 'How could you possibly lay down the rules to such an august body as The Royal Society?' He then explained this was the world's most lofty scientific institution; that it was a huge honour to be asked to chair anything there. I obviously had no idea – which just goes to show how ignorant I was in such matters.

The debate and the day went magnificently. I was chauffeured from and to the train station and subsequently received an invitation to a black-tie summer soiree at the opulent Royal Society headquarters at Carlton House Terrace.

It was a totally lavish affair and I rose to the occasion

– fabulous dress, the works. Not likely to be repeated, I thought, so let's make the most of this.

And I did! I bought an exquisite long gown, and turned up at the venue bang on time. I didn't want to miss anything. Everyone was invited who had given something to the Royal Society that year. The TV presenter Adam Hart Davis delivered a lecture on Sir Isaac Newton in the library. Marquees were set up on the rooftop terrace overlooking The Mall. We must have looked a remarkable sight, men and women resplendent in formal evening dress. It felt rather like being in a film. The food was incredible, in taste and presentation. I marvelled at the fact that I was here among all these scientists who had contributed so greatly to society. All I had done was chair a debate session on genetic testing for breast cancer.

HELEN AND BECKY

My cousin Jennifer's daughter, Helen, had tested positive for the fault in BRCA1. We had all undergone our genetic tests at the same time when Helen was 21. Now, eight years later, she decided perhaps it was time to discuss her future. She attended Gareth's clinic, and underwent a routine examination and mammogram. What happened next was a jolt to us all. Helen had blithely assumed that 30 was the age to start worrying. We all believed that up until that point she was unlikely to develop any ill effects from this faulty gene. How wrong we were.

Helen was found to have a two-inch cancerous lump in her right breast. This was such a shock to her as she had not felt anything at all. Now she was faced with the ordeal of surgery and everything that went with it. The surgeons were taking no chances. She had an immediate mastectomy on that breast, followed by radiotherapy and an intensive course of chemotherapy. She dealt with it amazingly well. As she said, her mum had survived; so must she. She decided to go ahead with preventive surgery on the other breast to reduce future risk.

We dealt with this as a family, in the way Helen wanted. She is a great personality and is likely to turn up with pink hair and trademark tangerine trousers, looking gorgeous. She thinks the world of her family and now, whilst battling with this disease herself, Helen's concern was for my daughter, Becky. Helen had managed to get on with her life by almost ignoring the implications, and I can quite understand why one would adopt this approach. Now Becky, aged 22, was suddenly plunged into a world of uncertainty. She had initially sailed along, expecting to go through her twenties without breast cancer rearing its ugly head, but Helen's case put a whole new aspect on the situation. Decisions that Becky had felt comfortable with, particularly while they were still in the future, were now very much upon us.

Becky had been with her boyfriend, Carl, for a number of years. He was well versed in all the family issues, and there was little Carl he did not know about our family's breasts. Nonetheless, Becky was concerned about how Carl would cope with her having a genetic test, which might force a decision on her at this stage. She needn't have worried one iota. Carl was totally at ease with the whole situation. For a young lad he was remarkably mature, his total adoration of Becky was evident to everyone. Carl encouraged Becky to take the test if and when she felt ready. This was an enormous relief to her. Along with countless others, Becky had the natural worry of the 'partner coping syndrome'.

I said very little to Becky. She knew she could ask for advice any time she wished. She had worked on the helpline at times, and was totally conversant with most of the facts. She had lived more than most in this faulty gene environment, having given interviews regularly since she was a child.

She had an appointment to see Gareth and discussed the testing at some length. Before she was allowed to take any test, rigorous psychological assessments were needed to ensure the patient could cope with the results. She went through her appointments then took the test. I went with her. By this time we had our own media circus in the form of the *Tonight with Trevor McDonald* crew. They were great. It always meant that we had company on every appointment too. Becky took the decision herself to allow in the film crew, and had great confidence in the producer and her 'angle'. I obviously left this to Becky, but I was happy to discuss any or all of it, which we did whenever Becky felt the need.

I'm unsure who was most nervous when we went back for Becky's results. If I'm honest, I think it was me, as we sat waiting in the small designated area for our appointment with Gareth. He, of course, was fantastic. He ushered us into his office and just got on with it. 'It's bad news I'm afraid,' were his exact words. He then proceeded to show us the evidence, that incomprehensible set of letters which mean nothing to the layman and everything to the knowledgeable expert.

I always describe a gene fault by drawing an analogy with a library. A single cell is the library. In the library there are several sections; the cell equivalent of those are chromosomes. Each chromosome is made up of thousands of genes (or books), and each one of those books (genes) contains thousands of words. Somewhere in the gene, or book, is a spelling mistake. It is a great way to understand the complexity of genetic testing. I imagine standing outside the British Library and being told, 'There's a spelling mistake in there.' Thus, genetic testing is not so simple until the spelling mistake is found in an affected family member. Of course, at the library, if you knew in which book, which chapter and which misspelt word you were searching for, it would be very easy to home in on that exact area and find it. And that is exactly the same with testing for genetic faults. Gareth has a fantastic attitude towards his patients. He treats people as if they might like to understand the details, which is wonderful; so much better than a blanket opinion.

The next step was for Becky to decide when – or indeed whether – to do anything at all with this news. She was pretty certain from the outset she would like to have surgery though, at her age, the reconstruction aspect was obviously of greater importance than it had been for me. She was booked to see surgeon Andrew Baildam. She asked Andrew his view on surgery at her age. He said the youngest breast cancer patient he had treated was aged 17. Becky needed no further ado. The operation was booked for January 2006, around six months later. Becky wanted to see pictures, to show Carl what she might look like. Unfortunately, these were not so easy to find. This was one thing Becky herself decided she must do after it was over. She wanted to have pictures taken and then make them available for display, so that others who were facing surgery might derive hope and encouragement.

Having the *Tonight* team with us made more of a meal of everything than perhaps would have happened otherwise. They had a programme to make though, and we were glad to co-operate. It was very nice too, for Becky to receive this attention. From start to finish, with genetic testing appointments, psychological assessments and visits to the surgeon, the timescale was just over a year. As the operation neared, I wondered how Becky would cope. One day she came in from her work as a local radio presenter. I was at the computer and she sat on my knee. 'Mummy, I'm scared,' was what she whispered. I told her that this was totally normal and reassured her she could back out if she wished. Inside though, my heart was breaking for her. She was my baby. When I went through surgery, I had been fine, but I was 37 years old, not 24.

Only a day or so later Becky returned.

'That's it,' she said. 'I can't wait now to get it over.'

She had read Caron Keating's story, and it had inspired her to march on. She would have done so anyway, but sometimes others' stories are such a help. Of course, this was the basis of the helpline. People felt empowered, and could relate to our pragmatism. It gave them the courage to follow their own hearts – so important.

We sped through the next week or so. I bought my daughter a teddy with matching dressing gown and slippers to accompany her to hospital. (Okay, so she was 24, but she was still my baby!) We drove to the hospital at Wythenshawe, where I stayed the night with her. The staff were marvellous.

After the *Tonight* team had left for their hotel, Becky and I wandered to the canteen. We had a meal and just tried to chat, both of us 'living' our own anxieties. I was trying desperately not to show mine, telling myself the operation was easy and non-invasive, and she was fit and young – all the logical reasons not to worry. By this time, I think Becky just wanted to move it all on, get it over and done with. I was with her all the way.

In the morning, Becky was first on the list. I was

allowed to accompany her to the pre-op room, where Andrew Baildam drew pictures of where any cuts might be. He had decided he could keep the scarring very minimal by making the incision around the areola of the nipple, then a small line down, rather like a question mark. He planned to take away as near to 95 per cent of the tissue as possible, leaving only a blood supply to the nipples, which Becky had chosen to keep. All the breast tissue would be scooped out and replaced with expanders. These were simple implants with a small 'port' to enable filling with a solution to grow the breast to the appropriate size; this would be required in small stages. Becky did not opt for any muscle being brought round from her back; just the implant under the chest muscle.

With this type of reconstruction, a trip to the hospital for further 'pumping up' of these expanding implants is required, usually about once a month or six weeks, depending on the individual. Once the required size has been reached, a simple operation is performed to remove these harder implants and replace them with the softer, more natural-feeling permanent silicone ones. There are so many different styles of reconstruction, using different types of implants to replace the lost breast tissue. Many surgeons opt also to bring a muscle round from the back, to give a natural feeling in addition to a small implant. Occasionally this is taken from the tummy. Mr Baildam favoured the simple silicone implant for Becky.

All went well. I sat in my room, waiting and waiting. Carl came over and waited too, neither of us saying very much. Halfway through the morning, one of the camera crew came into my room to film my reactions. This was a massive relief: the camera crew were able to give me an update, and evidently the whole process was going extremely well. I started to relax.

Around lunchtime we were summoned. Becky was now in the recovery room. When we went in, she opened her eyes and gave a huge drunken smile. She said she felt totally sloshed, inebriated, smashed. Her speech slurred in precisely that way. She looked down at her chest and saw the wonderful result already apparent. I was at this point overcome with emotion. I was so relieved; it was ridiculous how tearful I was.

Meanwhile, Becky had everyone in hysterics. She was busy showing her new breasts to anyone who would look. The success of the operation was displayed to the trolley porters, the cleaners, any passing nurse – everyone had to have an eyeful. When we got back to her room she was supposed to rest. You must be joking; she was awake in a state of euphoria!

Gareth popped in to see her after his clinic and even he wasn't exempt from the display.

'Look Gareth,' Becky said proudly. Gareth tried to resist the invitation, but Becky wasn't taking no for an answer. The new front-fastening nightdress was undone at the speed of light by the impatient Becky, delighting in showing off her new wares. Gareth too was delighted that his youngest patient to elect for genetic testing and risk-reducing surgery was happy. The operation was a success.

Joking apart, the results were truly amazing – and immediate. Becky's new breasts already had some shape. Mr Baildam had managed to get about 100 mililitres of saline into each expander immediately, which gave her a great shape and a cleavage.

Becky came home after five days. I think day two in hospital was her lowest point. The adrenalin that had kicked in with such verve became depleted. It was probably the body saying, 'Look here, Becky, we need to get some rest.' I knew she would be restless fairly quickly so she commandeered me into an expensive trip to Hobbycraft, getting me to spend pounds on beads and glitter, flowers, clay, enamel, paints, books. You name it, we bought it. I think some of the projects were started; most of them are still in boxes, incomplete.

Becky's friends, and the listeners to her morning radio programme, sent hundreds, maybe even thousands of messages. I had known that as soon as her strength was up, there would be no stopping her. She is so similar to me in so many ways, and of course she was even younger than I was. Remembering how euphoric I had become after my own surgery, I had expected a similar result for Becky. Very soon the 'craft department' was abandoned for more exciting exploits. For a start there was a new cleavage to sport. Becky was very clear that her surgery had been to rid her of as much risk as possible, but you cannot help being delighted if the end result is so much better than expected.

No one can believe Becky's surgery. It is magnificent, yet she has virtually no natural breast tissue left at all. Mr Baildam has since said how delighted he is with the result, and has reassured us that most of the actual breast tissue had been scraped away. The man is a genius, and we hope that more surgeons will emulate this level of care and detail. The *Today* team were delighted with their filming. They continued to follow her progress and keep in touch, but in reality the filming was all but over. We organised a party for family and friends to celebrate, and conclude the filming. Life then returned to normal, until the programme was edited and the next round of publicity was put into action by the *Tonight* press office.

Life moved on. The programme was widely viewed, which made the helpline enormously busy. I wasn't worried about that, we expected it, and it had been the main reason for allowing any filming at all. The overwhelming viewer reaction was that people found Becky's story inspiring. Such a young girl so stoically accepting her fate. There were no histrionics, no 'why me's, just rational plans to be made and events to be dealt with in the best way possible. Chris was extremely supportive of Becky, although he stayed out of the picture and all the filming. Becky, like me, had been incredibly lucky. Lucky to have this choice available, and even luckier to have such a magician as her surgeon.

We made great friends with many of the people who contacted us. Some you get to know more than others, perhaps because of their sheer need.

JILL

It was through the helpline that I had the great pleasure of meeting Jill and her delightful family.

Jill had contacted us after seeing Becky's documentary. Her younger sister, Suzanne, had recently died from breast cancer, and Jill's father had been told almost a year later that he had passed the gene on to his daughter. The turmoil in the family was so terribly painful; even just to hear their story made you really want to reach out and hug them. Jill was now facing the prospect of her own future which, before seeing Becky's documentary, had seemed bleak. She had been offered a genetic test which had just seemed to her to be a potential delivery of a death sentence. Seeing the documentary and the helpline number had galvanised Jill into a more positive approach. We could still hear the desperation though, so then and there we invited the family for lunch to meet Becky, and to take a look at what could be the worst case scenario.

Jill and her mum promptly took us up on this. Jill and Becky were not a million miles apart in age, and had by now become firm telephone friends. I remember so clearly everyone sitting at my kitchen table, eating lunch and talking of their traumatic years, of coping with the harrowing death of their youngest daughter and sister. Jill showed me a photo of Suzanne in hospital only days before her death. She was bloated from the steroids she was pumped full with. They related the story of Suzie's diagnosis, treatment, relapse and death.

Margaret, Jill's mum, was battling her grief within herself. Her husband would hardly talk about things at all, and she felt as if she was living in a vacuum. Margaret was now clearly hugely concerned for Jill, and immensely saddened that her husband would not talk about this. Richard was not with us, but immediately my heart went out to him. Not only had he lost his 31-year-old daughter, but a year after her death he was told they had found the mutation in Richard's side of the family. His mother had developed and died from ovarian cancer. I was not surprised that he couldn't talk about this. Everything that Jill had said about her dad strongly indicated a caring, loving, family man. I tried gently to say to Margaret that he had the toughest job of anyone. Jill's own position could be resolved fairly easily. By this time Becky's famous breasts had been on display for Jill and Margaret to inspect, prod, and generally marvel over.

'If this is the worst case scenario for me,' said Jill, 'I can cope!'

I talked with Margaret about her relationship with her husband or, rather, Margaret talked to me. There were many tears shed over that lunch, but both Jill and Margaret declared how much better they felt afterwards. I hoped that Margaret would understand that Richard's reticence was in no way a reflection of their relationship, but just something that was far too painful for him to express. I suppose these things are easy to see from the outside, and I had had the benefit of taking hundreds of calls in a similar vein. The feeling of parental guilt is one of the big issues which is rarely addressed.

Over the next few weeks and months we saw Jill several times; we were only around an hour and a half's drive from Leeds where she lived. When a man called Simon Towers wrote a book about Becky and her story, calling it *No Big Deal*, Jill came to the book launch.

Jill wrote to the Department of Health about her experiences, and expressed concerns for the existence of the helpline with the ever-increasing difficulties in obtaining funding:

My younger sister, Suzanne, was diagnosed with breast cancer at the age of 29 and died of metastasis to the pleura and brain just two years later at the age of 31. She worked for the NHS as a Medical Secretary at Leeds General Infirmary and St. James's Hospital, Leeds, and had the best care at the time. Unknown to the consultants at the time, she carried the BRCA1 faulty gene which she inherited from my dad, we now know. Not only are we still in complete despair and shock of what happened, the nightmare goes on! I am now currently waiting for the test.

I have to say, that up until the point of finding the phone number for the National Hereditary Breast Cancer Foundation I have not been able to imagine a future since seeing Suzanne die the way she did. The fear has been indescribable.

Wendy and her daughter Becky have been there for me every step of the way. So far, with their guidance, I am managing at last to dare think I can have a future. Not only have they spent time giving me the information and help I need, they have supported my mum and even given a lifeline to my father who has been struck down with so much guilt since. So in one family alone affected, this service is helping many members of the family including aunties, cousins, uncles, etc . . .

When I first went for genetic counselling, I felt so isolated and alone. The day I contacted Wendy I started to get my life back. Wendy could sense that I was not coping at all with the news of the BRCA1 gene fault in our family and went out of her way to provide lunch for myself and my mum to discuss the important information and knowledge she has gathered over the years. This was INVALUABLE! I have since met with other women in my area who have been through and are going through gene testing and just look at the Breast Cancer Forums!

There are so many women in their 20s, 30s and 40s all desperate for information about a gene fault running in their families and the one thing they all come back to is, 'How helpful and comforting it is to know that there is always somebody on the end of the phone to talk to' regarding the helpline. I had to be referred to the Psychosocial Oncology Team earlier this year to try and get me to the point of being able to take the test and 'then do something about it' and I know that the doctor I have been seeing has taken great interest in the National Hereditary Breast Cancer Foundation and has been able to pass on this information to help other patients. I have managed to get to the point of testing myself with Wendy's support, therefore I now do not need the resources of the Psychosocial Oncology Team.
Jill

Of course, this spoke volumes. The Department of Health was to receive many such letters from patients and geneticists, all of whom recognised the tremendous value of the service.

Jill took the genetic test. The whole family waited with bated breath until the day of the results. The day before, Jill and her mum came over again for lunch, more for moral support and another dose of positive thinking I guess. I could obviously in no way influence the test result, just make it more bearable. I recognised though that this lovely, pretty girl was now more in control of herself. She was totally decided on her course of action and could deal with the prospect of a faulty gene. Of course, our job is *not* to persuade people to have their breasts removed, but to realise that it is an acceptable option.

Jill's result was negative. For a time no one could believe it. Jill's mum and dad, whilst now prepared for the fact that the fault need not be a death sentence, were obviously over the moon with the good news. Maybe, just maybe, this family could piece itself together again. I hoped so. Nothing could ever bring Suzanne back. Nothing could, or should, wipe away the memories of that painful ending to such a short life, but hopefully a light was now glimmering at the end of this dark tunnel.

Only a couple of months later I received some wonderful news from Jill. She had been trying for a baby for several years, and had now just discovered she was pregnant. She also said that not a day went by without her thinking about Becky and me, yet I almost felt we did nothing in particular. We just talked naturally about our own situations, which I think is probably the most effective part of this whole process. We are so positive about our experiences, yet we empathise and understand the doubts and fears. Little Eloise was born into a happier family who now dote on her. Christmas is still a trial for Richard and Margaret.

Margaret, Richard and Jill are now training to work on the helpline. Margaret and Richard are such an asset, giving our callers a perspective, as only those who have lived through this could do.

There are so many remarkable stories that it is very hard to single them out. Each one has a common theme, but its own personal slant. I cannot possibly tell you about all of the thousands of calls; it's hard to remember exactly the details of each individual's worries. I have limited myself to telling you about those stories from people I have actually met up with, as they remain in my memory longer. I can usually recall every element of our conversations as I become involved with everyone in a deeply personal way. If I didn't care so much, I would not be doing the job. When you empathise so profoundly with each and every scenario, it is hard not to become a leaning post, but I am still grateful every day that I had the courage to fly in the face of the Doubting Thomases. The testimonials on our website just make such heartrending reading.

SARAH

Sarah contacted me a few times by email and then by telephone. Her troubling genetic history was through her father's side of the family. Her situation is similar to Jill's, but with the difference that, while it was clear there was a genetic fault in the family, her defective gene could not be located. Either it was in a previously undetected gene, or it was a mutation or deletion in one of the known genes, but not evident using current technology. Either way, Sarah faced a decision based on uncertainty as to whether she in fact carried a fault.

Eventually I arranged to meet Sarah at Manchester after a meeting I had to attend at the Genesis Breast Cancer Prevention Centre.

We sat for around two hours in the cafe, picking on sandwiches, chatting away endlessly. Sarah's email says more than I could ever describe:

Hi Wendy,
I want to thank you from the bottom of my heart for the help and advice you gave to me and my husband Tony yesterday. As you know, I lost my sister to breast

cancer four years ago and my family are devastated. My sister was 27 when she was first diagnosed with breast cancer and she was extremely fit and healthy. She sadly lost her battle at the age of 30. Everyone in my family is struggling to come to terms with the loss of my sister and the pain and suffering she went through. My dad most of all is overwhelmed with guilt as it is through his side of the family that the faulty gene has been passed down. As you know, my sister had a genetic test shortly before she died which revealed she did not have either BRCA1 or 2, but Professor Gareth Evans has said her cancer was due to an unknown faulty gene as other family members like my dad's mum, died of breast cancer in her 30s. As it is an unknown gene I can't have any genetic testing and I'm in limbo.

I have two very young children and my ultimate fear is leaving my children motherless when I have the chance to do something about this. I have had a mammogram and I'm waiting for the MRI screening. So far everything is clear which is good, but although screening can detect a cancer at an early stage it does not prevent it. As well as the sadness of losing my sister both me and my family are frightened that the same thing could happen to me. For the last few years I have been thinking a lot about having preventative surgery but both me and Tony had many questions and concerns.

When we met you yesterday, for the first time, I felt so at ease. You are such a kind and caring person that I feel I have known you a while. Both Tony and I felt really comfortable talking to you and you put our minds at rest. When I went home yesterday I was buzzing, as you have no idea how much you have helped me. I've been into work today and I'm still buzzing!

One of my concerns about having surgery was how

my dad would deal with it and would he feel bad that this is what I'm going to do. As you suggested, I spoke to my mum and dad when I got home and told them my decision to have surgery and rid our family of this fear. It's my decision and I really want to do this. What can I say? My mum and dad feel such relief as we can look forward to living our lives as we should. I know there will always be a possible risk to my children but there will be at least 20 years before we need to worry. By that time they may have found our faulty family gene and cancer could be a thing of the past!!

As an NHS medical professional, I explain facts and figures to patients on a daily basis, to allow them to make an informed decision (as we cannot influence a patient's decision). And although you did not influence my decisions, meeting you yesterday and looking at your website has helped me immensely. Not only have my family and I benefitted but I have a good friend who is a physiotherapist and treats a lot of ladies who have had mastectomies. She has used your website a lot to help her with the treatment of these ladies and been able to pass on the details of your helpline to many others. I'm sure without a doubt that many allied health professionals could benefit from meeting you and Becky and learning about the good work you both do.

Thank you once again, will keep in touch,
Sarah (North Manchester) x

SUE

Sue contacted the helpline *after* she had undergone two operations for her elective mastectomies. She had chosen to have the fat and muscle tissue from her tummy used to create the newly reconstructed breasts. Things had not gone well; further operations were pending to put everything right. Sue wrote to us and we responded.

I didn't hear from Sue again for a year or so. She told me that she had now undergone five different operations to try to fix the problems that had occurred. Eventually the surgeon had had to replace the right breast tissue with an implant. This had slipped and Sue was now in a terrible situation. She could not wear anything other than her work tunic as she had one breast a good four to five inches below the other, misshapen and completely misplaced, and her surgeon had now given up. I felt so dreadfully upset for her. She was at her wit's end. Her daughter was getting married soon – finding an outfit was practically impossible.

I suggested to Sue that perhaps Becky's surgeon, Andrew Baildam, would be best placed to rectify things for her. I attempted to arrange a referral to this genius man. Sue was so grateful, for what were only a few well-chosen phone calls I made.

As the time for Sue's appointment grew nearer, she became more and more terrified, paranoid that Andrew would take one look at her and declare, as her current surgeon had, that there was nothing he could do. I promised to meet Sue and accompany her, for support. If I had offered her a lottery win, her gratitude could not have been greater. Somehow or other, I now had the status of friend, adopted mum, and sister all rolled into one.

We met up at Andrew Baildam's consulting rooms, where he welcomed us both in his quiet, warm manner. He spent about half an hour talking to Sue, listening to the story of all her failed surgical procedures. I sat there quietly, also listening to all that she had endured. Andrew then took Sue behind a curtain to examine her. The intensity of the silence spoke more than any words he could have uttered. His professional code and conduct was impeccable. He calmly explained how he would have to proceed in order to rectify things. Eventually, after a lengthy examination and discussion, Andrew came out from behind the curtain. Before she got dressed, Sue called me and asked me if I would like to see the damage. This poor, poor girl! Her left breast was reasonable, but the right side revealed no anatomical resemblance to a breast. It now had the appearance of an enormous flattened bread cob, situated in totally the wrong place. I couldn't believe my eyes.

Sue's gratitude to Andrew was so touching, as was his compassion for her. I, like an idiot, felt tears welling that I could not stop. Once again, a possible happy ending was in sight.

Only a few days later, Sue wrote the most touching email to Vicki, our lovely volunteer Girl Friday:

Hi Vicki
Wendy became my saviour and my best friend all in one day of meeting her. I was at my lowest ebb. When I used the helpline to speak to Wendy I couldn't see any way of my life getting any better. I came off the phone feeling a lot better and Wendy got the ball rolling for me to meet my new surgeon.

Then I met Wendy. She came with me the day I went to meet my surgeon. She travelled over an hour and a half to be with me to give me support. This is the kind of woman Wendy is. She is great and brilliant and a friend to everyone who needs her. Wendy deserves so much more than words can say, but she is an incredible woman whom I've come to care for so very much. LOVE YOU WENDY.
Regards
Sue xxx

If ever there was a reward for doing this job, here it is. I am no saviour; I am just someone who is motivated to put injustices to rights. This is what drives me. The job is a total pleasure; everyone wants to be needed and useful. I know I do, and the appreciation I receive is simply the icing on the cake.

Sue has now had the first phase of her corrective surgery. I met her one lunchtime a few weeks after her operation and she showed me the result. I was astounded! The slipped breast had been perfectly re-sited and her other breast matched. It was remarkable. We hadn't any idea how successful this might be, but seeing this, I was overwhelmed with gratitude towards Andrew Baildam. Sue was bubbling and chatting away, confident, happy and so thankful – such a change in personality – and my reward was to behold the incredible result after the disaster she had been left with. Sue continues to send me messages and emails, just general family chit-chat. She will soon go back into hospital to have nipples made and tattooed. This sounds impossible, but is extremely clever. In exactly the correct place, the surgeon puckers the skin to make a nipple, and several weeks later the colouring of the areola is tattooed on. It's very difficult to tell in most instances as it looks so real.

Sue's cousin Andrea has now had a similar operation, despite resistance from her mother. Her mother was so strongly against this operation, that eventually Andrea had to make a choice. Her husband, however, was extremely supportive of this action, and Andrea decided the rift was worth it. Why shouldn't her mother want her to take every action possible to save her life? Throughout this traumatic time, Andrea and I were in close contact. I was particularly careful not to influence her in any way, but she was resolved. She did however need a friend, and that was just what I became. Many times we would chat online if Andrea was disturbed in the night and she saw I was logged on. It would probably be desultory conversation, but each time Andrea said she felt less anxious about the whole thing and would go to bed more relaxed. Everyone has different needs, and everyone should have the opportunity to talk to someone who understands and listens to them. Cousins Sue and Andrea both keep in touch regularly, updating me with their progress.

NICE GUIDELINES

It eventually became apparent to me that, in the early days, my role had not just been in supporting and enabling the patient, but in raising knowledge, education and awareness of the issues in any way I could. Now, it appeared that my time was being used wastefully, explaining to GPs one by one that yes, the gene can be passed down the male line, and yes, Mrs X would qualify for referral to genetic services. Not that I minded, but how much better it would be, I thought, if there were guidelines from the National Institute for Health and Clinical Excellence, more generally known as NICE, on criteria for referral. Surely this would be the best way of tackling the inequality in referrals? Fairly soon, NICE decided this was indeed an area which needed investigating, and I was invited onto the committee as one of the lay members; a patient advocate.

From the outset I was extremely impressed with the way the committee was selected. We were all bound to reveal a taped declaration of conflict of interest which was marvellous I thought – tackling any possible corruption or vested interests before they occurred. The structure was excellent, as was the education on how the process worked.

I think we had about ten meetings before the Guidelines were published. Everybody had their specific task; the other two patient advocates and I were mainly to oversee the literature and ensure the needs of patients were being considered. Of course, I was bound to fulfil that role to the best of my ability. This was exactly what I had been after for such a long time: laid-down criteria, decided by experts in the presence of health economists to ensure equity. Brilliant, and just what we needed. What three per cent of the female population, who are recognised as being at 'at least' moderate risk (one in six – one in four lifetime risk) needed.

One of the points raised by Michelle Barclay from Breakthrough Breast Cancer, was the value of and need for helplines such as mine. This was echoed by the rest of the Guideline Committee, and I was gratified that these professionals all recognised the real value patients found from this contact. It is one thing for everyone to write letters of support, but quite another having professionals suggest that this was a NICE requirement. I was very glad to have official recognition of the value of peer support and to have someone who understands the difficulties in explaining everything to well-meaning colleagues and friends.

The NICE guidelines are based on an evaluation of all the evidence of effectiveness of clinical trials into treatments at differing levels of risk. It gives a sound basis for criteria for referral to specialist services, enabling consistency of treatment around the country. Who should receive extra surveillance or adjuvant therapy, what type, how frequently, and so on. A patient booklet is available on 'Women with Breast Cancer in the Family – Understanding NICE Guidance'. As of this book going to press, guidelines are being updated.

PRIMARY CARE TRUSTS

Had I realised what the 'peer support' element in the NICE Guidelines would mean to my helpline, I'm not sure how I would have reacted. Talk about riddles! Here is the classic.

The Department of Health had initially given me a Section 64 grant to run the helpline. Section 64 grants are for novel projects that complement the services already available through the NHS. In 2006, when NICE guidelines were published, I was told this could no longer be considered as a 'novel project'. Ten years of Section 64 funding was apparently remarkable, but it was intended solely for novel projects and this service could no longer be classed as that. It was now a service required by NICE as the Guidelines said. The Cancer Policy Team Leader at the Department of Health told me it was now the responsibility of PCTs to fund this.

'PCTs? What on earth are those?' I asked.

'Oh, they are the old Health Authorities,' he replied. 'They are now called PCTs – Primary Care Trusts.'

I contacted my own PCT (Derbyshire County) in

order to obtain a list of these bodies. David Sharp, the Head of Commissioning, invited me to meet him. He agreed that Derbyshire would host the service for the year 2007/08. They would pay me the full amount, then they would invoice out to other PCTs as each individual PCT needed to pay its portion of the fee for our service. This was duly put in place, with Derbyshire sending an invoice to every PCT for £425. I blithely went along with this arrangement, grateful that Derbyshire County PCT should have taken this on.

A while later, I received a call from Derbyshire PCT, asking me to please call Leicester PCT to explain what service was provided.

Of course, I was delighted to do this. Everyone I had ever spoken to always thought the helpline was fantastic. By now I was used to being praised, cosseted, loved and admired for this and had no reason to be concerned. I contacted Leicester and, indeed, they agreed the service was great. This happened with several more PCTs, and then Derbyshire dropped the bombshell on me: hardly any of the PCTs other than those I had spoken to, they told me, had paid. In fact, some had written to Derbyshire and downright refused. This was a huge worry. I desperately wanted Derbyshire PCT to continue funding me, but they were not likely to do so without co-operation from the other Trusts. And indeed why should they? Why should Derbyshire prop up the rest of the country? I could quite understand their difficulties.

I took on the task of trying to get Derbyshire's money in for them. Not easy, but I persisted. I was quite sure if I managed to speak with the right person, they would see all the evidence for themselves. The value for money, sound business case, and of course the brilliant testimonials from both professionals and patients would do the trick, I was certain.

For the most part, I managed to get Derbyshire's money in for them, but the cost to the PCT of providing me with up-to-date spreadsheets was greater than the actual money being recouped. I had a growing feeling of doom about this and, just as I anticipated, David Sharp wrote to me, stating he was very sorry but he could not continue the arrangement the following year. Recovering the money from the other Health Authorities had proved to be too problematic.

Oh dear, oh dear, oh dear.

Nothing for it, I must do it myself. So, with customary gung-ho, I invoiced each PCT. As a goodwill gesture I lowered the cost per PCT by £10. What an idiot! In fact, a few of these commissioners would just have viewed this with disdain for the most part. To be fair, I initially made good relationships in the PCTs – until I encountered Hull . . .

Having taken the bull by the horns, I researched the format required for invoicing PCTs, the various documents they might need (service level agreements, business case, governance document and professional endorsements ad nauseam). These I provided in spades. Professor Gareth Evans gave me an Evaluation and Support document, as follows.

Central Manchester and Manchester Children's University Hospitals

NHS Trust

Prof. Gareth Evans: Chair NICE GDG

Consultants:

Prof D Donnai	Dr B Kerr
Dr H Kingston	Prof G Black
Dr D Craufurd	Dr K Metcalfe
Prof G Evans	Prof D Trump
Dr J Clayton-Smith	Dr W Newman
Dr F Lalloo	Dr K Chandler

Consultant Genetic Counsellor: Mrs L Kerzin-Storrar
SCMO Genetic Register: Dr E Howard

Regional Genetic Service
St Mary's Hospital (SM2)
75 Hathersage Road
Manchester M13 0JH
UK
Tel: +44 161 276 6206
Fax: +44 161 276 6145

To whom it may concern

Hereditary Breast Cancer Helpline

The Helpline performs a vital service which has been used by thousands of women and reduces workload to the NHS. There is NO equivalent of this and existing lines at CANCER Backup, CR-UK, Breast Cancer Care and Breakthrough do NOT give the expertise afforded by the HBCH. GPs and genetic services have benefited from the improved patient information and appropriate reassurance to those not at risk. NICE guidance on Familial Breast Cancer requires and supports the use of such a helpline. The Manchester Regional Genetic Service uses the Helpline for women who attend, but PCTs are saved substantial sums on women who are appropriately reassured that they do not need specialist referrals.

Below is a list of the benefits of the service:

Well established helpline run for 13 years by a patient, but with general respect and support from the medical profession/genetic community. Prides itself in non-directional information resource for women.

Only Helpline open 24 hours per day, 365 days per year.

Still believed to be the only one of its kind in the world.

Huge database of women prepared to talk to others of their experiences with hereditary breast cancer issues.

Keeps abreast of all new or ongoing trials/treatments etc. and can provide information on these.

Used regularly by GPs as a resource facility i.e. nearest Genetic Centre, criteria for referrals etc. although NICE guidelines have recently been issued to assist them in this. Also used as point to refer women whose history is unclear, or to refer women who wish to chat to others about their dilemmas. It has been abundantly clear over these last few years that many women have found speaking to this Helpline a very empowering experience. Many have felt isolated, and having the facility to speak to others has been invaluable for them.

Helpline represented on NICE committee, MRC funded MARIBS trials.

Lobbies insurance industry regarding genetic testing

Complete understanding of such issues as Patents, and, from the outset, has been instrumental in helping ensure that genetic testing remains legal and available in the UK.

Helpline shown on all media (TV, radio, papers)

Wendy Watson or her daughter spend time explaining to women who appear to not have a significant family history how the genes work and assists them in further researching their family histories on BOTH sides to ensure that there are no other cases and to help them feel genuinely reassured.

Helpline number available in every GP surgery, NHS direct, and widely on the net.

Yours sincerely

Professor D Gareth Evans MD FRCP
Consultant in Medical Genetics and Chair of the NICE GDG on familial breast Cancer

I badgered the poor Cancer Policy leader at the DoH for a letter.

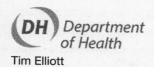
DH *Department of Health*

Tim Elliott

Team Leader
Department of Health
Cancer Policy Team
Wellington House
133-155 Waterloo Road
London
28th July 2008

To whom it may concern

Dear Colleague

Hereditary Breast Cancer Helpline

The Hereditary Breast Cancer Helpline was founded in 1996 by Wendy Watson with a Section 64 project grant from the Department of Health. The Department renewed the grant for ten years as Wendy's work was important and valued, but it became inappropriate to keep supporting the helpline through the Section 64 scheme. It is for Primary Care Trusts, working in partnership with their Strategic Health Authorities, local service providers and stakeholders to provide services for their local populations, including for women who are worried about their familial risk of breast cancer.

The helpline has provided an invaluable service to thousands of women over the years, and is supportive of the implementation of the NICE guideline Familial Breast Cancer (2006).

Wendy's commitment to the helpline and the thousands of women she helps is outstanding, and she is well respected in the genetics community. We wish Wendy every success in attracting the modest funding she requires to maintain this valuable service.

Yours sincerely

Tim Elliott
Team Leader: Cancer Screening and Male Cancer
Cancer Policy Team

This letter was easy for Tim Elliott to provide. He had already suffered under an avalanche of letters and emails from previous helpline users, ladies who were distressed, annoyed, angered and disturbed over funding issues in the past. He had received them all, and had been left in no doubt as to the enormous benefits of the service. He had equally to deal with me. I do give the poor chap his due – he coped with everything very professionally. Not once did I manage to cajole, wheedle or threaten any opinions from him. He upheld the civil service code to the bitter end, not even faltering over the more extreme cases. He coped with me in floods of tears at each injustice, every time I had to listen to a PCT or cancer network say how they didn't value the service. I was so hurt and upset. I had imagined that the views of patients and clinicians, all of whom had made such a fuss about me, would be similarly viewed by the fund holders. Tim had the perfect solution: 'go and have a cup of tea'. Very British, but it worked. Who on earth else could I moan at? Well done, and thank you, Tim!

Hull PCT wrote me a letter. The rough gist of it was that they did not want this service and would not pay last year, this year or in future years, so don't bother them again. I was repeatedly told that they already had this service available locally. Of course, I naturally asked them for the contact details, knowing full well this could not possibly be true. Eventually, after much deflection I was given the contact details of the Chair of the Patient Involvement Group.

A lovely older lady, Susan Raettig, Chair of the Hull and East Riding Patient Involvement Group, told me all about this latest news from Hull PCT. They had given me Susan's details stating she was involved with patient support. I contacted Susan and started to explain why I was calling. She was astounded. She told me they had nothing like this service at all in Hull. The group, of which she was Chair, was a general cancer group. In fact, I would go as far as to say that Susan was annoyed. To have given her details out and to claim she provided this service was ridiculous but she said, 'This is typical of our PCT, they have only just bought a yacht for nearly half a million pounds.'

'A yacht?' I exploded.

'Oh yes,' she said. 'For socially disadvantaged youngsters, aimed at providing them with the necessary skills to go out and get a job. Help them learn to value their lives better, which may have a favourable impact on their future health.'

I had now heard it all. I took this up with Alan Johnson, MP for Hull, who was also the Health Minister. I wrote faithfully the pages of emails recounting the story, the responses from the PCT, and the final denouement of the infamous yacht. Eventually, after a fairly long wait, I received a response from him. Not one I was happy with. He said it was up to each PCT how it spent its money for its 'local populations'. I have put those two words in quotes as they were to haunt me for the next two years. I even wrote to the Care Quality Commission and parliamentary ombudsman – all replied with the same mantra about 'local need' and being up to each PCT. My hurt and upset turned to anger at the injustice of it all

By now, we had the biggest pile of nonsensical excuses for not paying this £422. I sent this list of excuses out to our ladies who have used the helpline repeatedly. I sent it to clinicians and politicians, newspapers, and members of the public. Everyone is appalled, yet who really can do anything about it? As of today, there is £80,000 owed to the helpline in unpaid invoices to the Health Service over the past three years. Perhaps I deserve a tiny rant, given I have to pick up all the pieces.

During this time, I made contact with several of my old school pals. We had a reunion which was fantastic fun. Those people know you in a way that others from your present life just don't. Whether that's a good thing or not is hard to say!

One of my good friends was a girl called Elaine. I also had another great pal called Mark. One evening, when we were about 18, Elaine and I were out at one of the usual haunts for us teenagers, a pub called the Bluebell in Long Eaton. Mark was also there, having a drink with a friend of his, Geoff Hoon. We all four got together, and Elaine and Geoff really hit it off. They eventually married, and have both blamed and credited Mark and myself for this chain of events. Geoff went on to become an MP, then an MEP, and eventually a Cabinet Minister. We had many laughs together that evening, marvelling at how, in our wildest dreams, none of us could have predicted our futures at that earlier stage of life.

Geoff knew all about the helpline and he had followed the story through the media. He gave the helpline number to a colleague of his, Andy Burnham, who was to become Health Minister, and whose wife had a similarly strong family history of breast cancer. Thus, one evening I received a call from this extremely pleasant and bright young gentleman. He detailed his wife's family history, clearly a very significant one, and we chatted for a good half-hour on all the options. He was very interested in my own story and how I had become so involved in all of this. I gave him all the details of his nearest Genetic Service, the name of the consultant and everything he needed to give to his doctor. That was it. He thanked me profusely and stated how helpful it had all been. I thought little more about this except for musing on how this breast cancer gene can just pop up anywhere. Neither fame nor fortune could influence or exempt us from the strongest factor of inheritance.

Much later, Andy Burnham said on camera how invaluable that call had been. How he had been depressed and very low over the whole situation, feeling that cancer was crowding in on them. His wife's mother and sisters all developed breast cancer at very young ages. That call to the helpline empowered them to move forward, to see just what could be done. He talked of just being an ordinary punter, and said how talking through this calmly with someone who had themselves experienced all these feelings, and totally understood, helped him see this in a different light. He said they would always be grateful for that. He effusively paid tribute to my dedication to helping others.

BECKY AGAIN

By 2007 Becky had well and truly come through all her operations. She now had two ambitions. Her number one priority was to start a gallery of photos of the operation for people to actually see what the results of the surgery look like. We also hoped to inspire other surgeons to live up to Andrew Baildam's magnificent work, and have already gathered some more wonderful examples from across the country. Yet we still hear and see some horror stories, so hopefully we are doing our bit here. If women can point out to their surgeons what *can* actually be achieved, then it has to be worth it. Of course, everyone knows the reason for going through with this operation is *not* to have a Hollywood-style boob job, but if surgeons can perform this, to quote Mr Baildam, 'To help women so they don't look as if they had been attacked by a tin-opener', then all to the good. Why not? Becky's gallery took off and has been used by thousands. Indeed, the personal stories and photos are just about the most important pages on our website.

Becky's other ambition was to try her hand fundraising for the Genesis Appeal, the charity we are aligned with. She came up with fantastic ideas, and her job at Peak FM helped her bring them to fruition. The Peak FM listeners had followed Becky's story throughout, which meant most of the people in the Chesterfield region knew her. She had gathered so much wonderful support from everyone. Becky raised almost £50,000 with her calendar and all her other ventures. The Genesis Appeal was extraordinarily grateful to her.

Eventually the difficulties with the helpline began to cause grave problems. We could not continue to pay even the small amount needed for salaries, and the situation was becoming desperate. We needed to train others to help, we needed to get leaflets printed and distributed. But there is only so much spare time available when you are running a busy 24-hour service.

Becky turned her attention to fundraising for the helpline. She held our first charity ball at Chatsworth House in March 2009. There I was to witness my fantastic daughter's capabilities. Right, before anyone thinks it, I am not biased, she just happens to be brilliant!

She had transformed the Carriage House Restaurant into the most glamorous venue imaginable, and sold out the event with no problem at all, thanks to Becky's popularity, both through her work and her friends. It was sheer fantasy, and pleasure. The lighting, the flowers, the fantastic band, fire-eaters, stilt-walkers, no holds barred. I received a standing ovation from the guests which took my breath away. I could scarcely believe all these plaudits were for me. Geoff Hoon was our guest of honour. He had done his research well, and his speech was incredibly moving. He referred to the colleague who had used the helpline a few months previously, and had confided how helpful it had been to speak with someone who understood. Becky raised a wonderful £8,000 profit from this event, which provided at least some of the contributions not forthcoming from the PCTs.

But life was getting sillier. I had naively thought that the views upheld by all clinicians, patients and well-known politicians would be warmly embraced by these NHS fund holders. I really believed those two strong letters written by the Chair of the NICE Guideline Committee, and the Head of Cancer Policy in the DoH would be gladly received as knowledgeable support for this service. To keep dealing with these curt refusals was very hard to take. The attitudes of these PCTs were worse than dismissive, and almost aggressive in some instances. Yet the clinicians were supporting us more than ever before, while the patients were desperately upset over the injustice as they saw it.

The Department of Health commissioned a review of needs and services. This review concluded that the Hereditary Breast Cancer Helpline was the only one that actually provided the essential support which their findings proved necessary. Even that was ignored by most PCTs.

I spoke with Mike Hotson at Leicester County and Rutland PCT, a Trust which had doggedly refused to pay from the start. He said that 'they' couldn't tell them what to do. Unfortunately, he was correct. The PCTs had the power to spend their money as they saw fit, even if that included £200,000 salaries, and yachts to benefit their 'local populations'. They were deemed the best judges of what might benefit us, the taxpaying population, as they had been given a mandate to this effect.

Leicester City, their counterpart, had always paid; in

fact, I had a contract with them until the end of March 2011. I'm sure it was not worth the paper it was written on; one day in spring 2010, I received a call from their contracts manager, Polly Whelby, to tell me that, due to government cuts, they had to cancel many of these contracts. To add insult to this injury, she wanted to meet me to discuss what impact it would have on my service by pulling the plug on the £8-per-week contribution they had been making.

I immediately asked, 'Well, I do hope you aren't expecting me to drive to Leicester in order to tell me you cannot now afford this £8 per week?'

'Oh no,' was the response, 'I will drive up to the Peak District to see you.'

I was now totally flabbergasted. If they needed the money that badly I could see no point in driving out here to waste even more. I did point out that so far there were no cuts at all to the frontline. The PCTs had received their standard 5.5 per cent annual increase that year, but they were supposed to cut their own management costs by 30 per cent. She had no answer to this, except to say, 'Do I take it you don't want me to visit you?'

Southampton wrote that they did not need this helpline service, as 'Patients in the city with a background of hereditary breast cancer are offered an MRI scan through the acute Trust on a recurring annual basis.' That was just so ill informed, I could scarcely believe it. How could someone who had so little idea of everything be making funding decisions? It seemed crazy to me. Apart from the fact that that wasn't the point, it was also untrue. Completely inept.

Plymouth's spokesman was clearly not a doctor as in GP or clinician. She stated that they wished to have an unpaid invoice credited off their system. They had a breast cancer support group. I tried to explain the differences, that these people do *not* yet have breast cancer; that it would be highly inappropriate from both sides for the 'at risk' people to attend a meeting, ostensibly for sufferers. It would exacerbate rather than alleviate their feelings of guilt. I was part way through my patient explanation when the doctor butted in saying, 'We will take this as a verbal credit note,' and put the phone down on me. By this time I had become used to this rudeness. If I ever asked a question, or had a response to theirs, and they didn't know what to say next, they always put the phone down. Rather cowardly, I thought.

East Lancashire PCT had the gall to instruct Professor Gareth Evans, Chair of the NICE Guideline Committee and, indeed, in charge of their local regional genetic service, to disregard his own guidelines. They instructed him *not* to give out the helpline number. He is the chief advisor! How on earth a mere PCT worker has the audacity to issue instructions to one of the world's most famous experts in the subject is beyond my, and everyone else's, comprehension.

The two neighbouring PCTS of Dorset and Bournemouth and Poole had a little collaboration. I was contacted one evening around 8.30 p.m. by the commissioner from Bournemouth and Poole PCT. She had rung just to tell me they were not paying this small invoice of £422. I was astonished to receive a call from a PCT at that time of night, but I nevertheless tried to explain the value as noted by the clinicians, patients and guideline committee. I could hear this was having no effect. I explained that the neighbouring PCT, Dorset, happily paid, and the cancer network was keen to have a consensus. I should have anticipated the next reaction – talk about setting myself up! The lady said she would ensure that Dorset didn't pay next year, then they would be the same.

I wrote this up and sent it to Dorset so they could expect this lobby by this commissioner. I always expect a backlash and I got it, but it appeared in an unexpected form. I received a call on the helpline from a lady with a fairly convoluted family history, more or less saying she hadn't been referred. I explained that with this history it might not be sufficient to access specialist services; however, I could help in further research of her family. The next question was on local support – was there any? Not that I knew of, I replied, but I would try to find out. I finally concluded that my initial suspicions that this was not a genuine call were confirmed when I started to give the address of the local regional genetic service in Southampton, and was curtly told, 'I know that address.' The parting question was very leading, 'Then I don't need to worry then?' I started to reiterate the need to further research the family before any certainty, and the call terminated. This just isn't the behaviour of the thousands of women I have received calls from over the years, not by a long way.

Just to be certain about the local support, I called Bournemouth and Poole PCT to see if there was any local support, and was given the number of their Health Information shop in ASDA. Obviously I called this and a very pleasant lady said yes, indeed, they did have details of support for Hereditary Breast Cancer. Could I hold on please? A minute later she returned with a leaflet from which she read out the details. My own! I asked if there was a local service, to which she replied, not that she knew of but ring this number (mine), they would be sure to know!

Lincolnshire PCT told BBC Radio Lincolnshire that they had never heard of the helpline, never heard of me, and never received an invoice. This was despite my being in receipt of numerous emails from them, with a substantial 'cc' list at their end. They then blamed the regional office and stated they would be discussing this at a regional meeting the following morning. Once again, I was appalled at the disregard for waste. There would possibly be £1,500 per hour spent sitting round that table discussing an £8-per-week helpline. The cost of the rent of the pot plant for the boardroom is four times that figure!

Eventually they came back to Radio Lincolnshire and told them they now had various family history clinics. Well, of course they do. And guess what, they *all* give out, as per NICE requirements, the helpline details.

Central and Eastern Cheshire just made life silly by agreeing to pay 90 per cent of the invoice on completion of an enormous questionnaire requiring details of calls, follow-ups, outcomes, etc. Unbelievable!

And so the list grew, each one seemingly vying with the other to produce the daftest excuse. I'm afraid the honours, though, went to Bromley. They came up with four different excuses, telling me of services they had, which on investigation, clearly did not exist. The first, Cancer – A Family Affair, was found to be an old web page, no longer functional. I left two messages on the helpline number given, neither of which elicited a response. I reported this fact back to Bromley, to which they gave the second excuse – they were looking into this provision within the next three months. To which I responded that if they had accepted the need was there, how about paying for last year? Also, how were they intending to set up this service for themselves? How would they find the personnel to fill the role? How especially could this be performed for little over £400 *per annum*? This received no response, until they had received further calls from me and letters from their geneticists stating what an invaluable service this was for their patients.

GUY'S AND ST THOMAS' NHS TRUST
October 2005

Dear Wendy
We are writing in support of your quest for continued funding of the Hereditary Breast Cancer Helpline. Many patients from the South East Thames region have made use of the support that this helpline has provided over the past nine years.

Having the opportunity to talk to someone who has experienced the difficulties of living with a family history of breast cancer, and who has personal knowledge of the dilemmas and issues involved in considering prophylactic surgery, is extremely important for many women in this situation. There is no other helpline service which enables women to talk to someone who can really understand what they are going through from a personal perspective. In addition, for many women it is reassuring to learn that you can put them in touch with other people locally to them.

For many years you have provided a 'patient's voice' in the developing field of cancer genetics and, at a time when service users' views are increasingly important in planning and implementing services, it is essential that your important work continues.

Please do not hesitate to contact us if there is any more we can do to help.

Yours sincerely
Ms Chris Jacobs   Dr Gabriella Pichert
GENETIC COUNSELLOR CONSULTANT IN CANCER GENETICS

....

Guy's and St Thomas' Hospital
Our department often refers patients to your helpline as another source for information and know many who have benefited from it. Patients' information needs are always met better by targeted information, but the choice on the internet is too vast to handle. The helpline acts as a personal filter to help patients in their search and we would want to see the support of your helpline continue in the long term.
Yours Sincerely
Dr Louise Izatt
Lead consultant in Cancer Genetics

These letters provoked an answer which took some comprehending. It seemed strange that there should be such antipathy. Each time I sent them correspondence that supported the service; but instead of being delighted, they searched for reasons to dismiss it as if it was a purpose, a rationale or a remit to find reasons *not* to fund. The next excuse was that they had the Chartwell Unit of Breast Care Nurses. I contacted this unit, and spoke with several very sympathetic nurses and receptionists, all of whom confirmed there was no helpline facility for genetic risk. They just simply did not have the time, nor were they set up to offer such a facility. I offered to send them some leaflets, which they gratefully accepted, and once again wrote to Bromley about their latest offerings.

The next response was from Clive Uren, the Chief Operating Officer, more or less stating they had wasted quite enough time on this. I rang him up, and waited. I received no response and so I rang again – and again. Eventually he condescended to call me back, and what happened next was the worst of all. He stated the reason (number five) they were not paying this £400 was because of advice from their Public Health Department, and the Cancer Network. Of course, I believed this, and set about making an appointment with their local Cancer Network Nurse Director, Tim Jackson. I genuinely believed he had instructed Bromley *not* to pay.

Following my presentation to the very nice Tim, and noting his obvious pleasure and support, I asked him why he had instructed Bromley not to pay the small invoice. Tim looked aghast and perplexed. He really didn't know what I was talking about. I told him what Clive Uren had said. Tim categorically denied even being asked the question by Bromley, let alone advising them not to pay.

By now I was totally incensed that a public servant, and one in such lofty authority, could cause such confusion. I was advised by the Department of Health to seek the assistance of the Strategic Health Authority. What are these, I wondered? Evidently they are similar to the regional Health Authorities, whose job it is to performance-manage the PCTs. Aha, I thought, I might just get somewhere. No such luck. A very accommodating young man, Dominic Harris, listened to this whole tangled tale of woe, and asked me to set it all out with all the accompanying correspondence. It took ages, but I did it. Once again, nothing happened.

I wrote a conciliatory letter to Bromley because, by this time, I had received numerous further calls from Bromley patients whom I just couldn't bring myself to direct to any of the fictional services Bromley claimed to host. The Director of Public Health wrote back, threatening me with legal action if I contacted Bromley again. Even the Department of Health forgot themselves momentarily, to express incredulity at the shenanigans I had to deal with.

Thankfully, throughout this, Becky continued fundraising. Events were developed all the time, from hog roasts to various smaller fun days. The generosity of some people is astounding. It upsets me every time I see an old lady reach into her bag and willingly donate a five-pound note towards a cause that the Health Service considers mandatory and essential, yet refuses to fund.

Becky gathered a willing band of helpers to assist her at these events; the publicity resulted in another growth spurt of callers using the helpline. Leaflets were sent to every Macmillan outlet and genetic service. Our army of supporters and helpers grew and grew. In fact, many of this group called themselves 'Wendy's Army'. They had photos done with this printed on. Astounding!

The first charity ball had been so successful that this soon became an annual event. Thus, in 2010, we invited Andrea and Rhonda, the two girls who were the whole reason this helpline started, to open the ball. They had now reached 40! This was a milestone which initially had seemed impossible for them to reach.

Their speech was incredibly moving. They spoke with frank passion about what the helpline had meant to them. One of the girls said, 'Since we have had our surgery we have been able to forget about breast cancer, and that's a nice place to be.' They paid tribute to the individualised manner in which each person had been treated. They described the benefits of the opportunity to speak to someone who understands from a personal perspective, and told of the battles with the doctors and Health Authorities, and the difficulties encountered when attempting to discuss their decisions with 'well-meaning friends, who all had their own opinions and were only too willing to share them'. They described the surgery, how they felt it to be necessary and the right move for them to make, but how it was 'a little bit less scary with Wendy just a phone call away'. I now have this very moving speech as the last track on my new fundraising CD, 'I Dreamed a Dream', available for a donation through our website. Both Andrew Baildam, the girls' wonderful surgeon, and I were close to weeping over the sincerity of their speech. In fact, the whole room was moved.

As this was a 'Hollywood' Ball, it gave us an opportunity to present awards to those people who had achieved so much for us, and in the whole field of hereditary breast cancer. Genesis Chairman Lester Barr read out a letter from Andy Burnham, Minister of Health at that time:

From the Rt Hon Andy Burnham MP
Secretary of State for Health

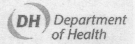

Richmond House
79 Whitehall
London
SW1A 2NS

Tel: 020 7210 3000

Ms Wendy Watson
Hereditary Breast Cancer Helpline
St Anne's Cottage
Over Haddon
Derby
DE45 1JE

Dear Wendy,

I am sorry not to be able to be with you at your wonderful Gala Ball at Chatsworth House and I hope that it is a really fabulous occasion for the National Hereditary Breast Cancer Helpline.

I am in great admiration of your work and determination over the years to bring this hugely important matter to public, medical and research prominence and your own courage to be the first woman in the UK to opt for a double preventative mastectomy.

The knowledge we now have of the genetic influence on breast cancer is highly significant and is, indeed, saving the lives of women of all ages by empowering them to understand their risk factors and take the decisions that are right for each one of them. Your work to support women and their families is tremendous and long may you continue.

Please pass on my very best wishes to all the people involved with this evening's ball and to all your workers and supporters.

With best wishes,

Andy

ANDY BURNHAM

AG 09.03

Our main sponsor, Adrian Fewings from Derbyshire Aggregates, said, 'Wendy is a star. She has worked so hard for years and put everything on the line just to be able to help others. What a fantastic lady. Derbyshire Aggregates are glad to have been able to help as sponsors of this brilliant and worthwhile cause.'

The auction proceeded to raise huge sums of money. Tea on the terrace at the Houses of Parliament, donated by Natascha Engel, our local MP, fetched a staggering £1550. This highlighted the wealth of support for this service, and the warmth with which everyone reacted. Natascha was totally astonished and told me that this was the talk of Westminster. No one could get over the fact that tea with Natascha had fetched this incredible sum. At least it revealed an awareness of the true depth of feeling the public had for this service.

Natascha then decided to take the situation on as a campaign. This help made a huge difference to me. I was incredibly relieved that someone with – hopefully – some influence, had recognised the desperate nature of the situation and wanted to help. I started to feel a little confidence returning.

I met Natascha at the station and we went for lunch. As I unburdened myself of all the story, the carry-ons that I had been dealing with, and the sheer intransigence of some PCTs and their attitudes towards me, it felt fantastic to have someone who was listening, who wasn't personally involved, yet who could actually do something. Natascha listened transfixed, and appalled. Although she was three assistants short, Natascha nevertheless put Lucy at my disposal to write to the non-paying PCTs, asking them to reconsider their non-payment decisions. I wasn't too optimistic. What regard would they have for an MP? Very little, I feared.

Unfortunately I was correct. Natascha continues to campaign on my behalf.

I now confided in a few people how desperate the situation really was, how dismissive the behaviour had been towards me from several of the PCTs, and how it was becoming increasingly difficult. Becky was so worried, bless her heart, that she and her friend Paula decided to perform a skydive parachute jump to help raise funds. That might not seem such a big deal, except that Becky has not only inherited my faulty breast cancer gene, but also my 'fear of flying' gene. Paula similarly has this fear, so this was even more of a major feat for them.

What was to happen then could not have been foreseen. Becky had said that both she and Paula were making up for some of the PCTs who refused to pay their small share of the helpline costs. No sooner had the girls made this known, than many of their friends, and other supporters from around Derbyshire, joined in. Pretty soon there were 36 people signed up to join in the venture! All were impassioned with the cause.

This gave me an idea; if they were 'jumping' to cover for PCTs who didn't pay their £422, why not each jump for a specific PCT and wear a T-shirt with the PCT name emblazoned across the front? Jumping for BROMLEY. Jumping for HULL. Jumping for EAST LANCASHIRE. And so on.

The more I thought about this, the more it appealed to me. I could write to the local papers with a press release and include, if they were willing, a local person who had used the service. This would raise awareness immensely. My brain was now in overdrive – why not hold another Hereditary Breast Cancer Awareness Week during which, as a finale, we would stage the mass skydive? It was an inspiration, and really funny.

Everyone seemed to like the idea. Vicki organised a meeting for those interested in either helping or skydiving. Brampton Manor Country Club in Chesterfield kindly hosted the meeting. The supporters packed the room. I told them of the plans, the publicity, the T-shirts and the silly reasons the health authorities came up with for not paying. I looked at the eager audience and could see the sheer disbelief on their faces. The story of Hull and its yacht, especially, gave everyone a renewed purpose and a local angle for their designated PCT.

During this period, Becky had cajoled a sponsored gazebo from Roger Stuart Racing and Printability. She also managed to obtain a vehicle to transport it around from T.C.Harrison. They loaned us a Ford Galaxy, logo-ed up with the helpline details. She had T-shirts designed with the helpline logo, and arranged a series of events more to raise awareness than funds. The evening before the very first of these events, I received a call from Dawn. It was around seven o'clock on the Friday evening.

DAWN

Dawn told me that her geneticist had given her the helpline number. Dawn had lived for the previous ten years with breast cancer featuring strongly in the family; her mum had died from the disease, and three weeks ago Dawn received the news that she had inherited the faulty BRCA2 gene. She was clearly extremely nervous and upset. She could see no future. She really felt she had been delivered a death sentence, with no way out. We chatted for around half an hour that Friday evening, Dawn telling me her story, punctuated with tears that she could not hold back. She told me that her eldest son had Asperger's Syndrome and saw things in black and white. I felt a huge empathy with her.

As Dawn lived fairly close by, in Rotherham, I suggested she might like to bring her sons to Chatsworth Rally Show the next day. We had our gazebo there and she could meet Becky and several others, all of whom would help her to see the normality of coping with this gene fault. Dawn was delighted and said she would come along at lunchtime. I really hoped she would; I believed that meeting us all might just help her feel more positive about the whole situation.

One thing Dawn told to me when she arrived was that, on the way over, her son Jordan had said, 'Mum, we're going to meet the lady who has saved your life.' He had looked everything up and come to the conclusion that his mother could now have preventive surgery, that she could see this as acceptable and normal rather than 'out of the question'.

Pretty soon, Dawn became one of the 'helpline team', attending events throughout the summer and feeling as if she had gained a family. That is a wonderful accolade to receive. She even signed up her long-suffering husband, Grant, for the skydive! Her own PCT, Rotherham, were one of those considering the helpline unnecessary. Grant gamely agreed to hurl himself from an aeroplane, and on his blog after the jump wrote, 'To misquote Winston Churchill, never in the field of Hereditary Breast Cancer has so much been done for so many by so few.' It spoke volumes. From that day onwards Dawn and her family looked forward to a brighter future. Dawn underwent her first operation to remove the ovarian cancer risk, and booked her second operation, the mastectomy, for May 2011. Between the two procedures, she kept herself occupied with organising a party in aid of the helpline. Her story captured people's hearts in her own locality, Rotherham.

JO

I was first contacted by Jo on the helpline while I was in Scotland, attending a meeting for Gengage. The conference was about women at moderate risk, but Gengage had been unable to locate a patient representative to speak at this meeting, and so I made the trip.

Jo told me that her mother and her aunt (her mum's sister) were both first diagnosed with breast cancer, aged 41 and 42 respectively, in 1990. Her mum had developed breast cancer again in 2002, but it was unclear as to whether this was a new primary or a recurrence. Now, in July 2010, she had developed breast cancer for a third time, but this was a new primary in the other breast.

Even before her mum had been diagnosed for the third time, Jo had already seen a genetic counsellor who decided that she did not qualify for genetic testing. In effect, she was told to wait and see if any other relatives developed the disease, even though there weren't many females in her family. However, with the diagnosis of a new primary in her mother, it was deemed a high enough risk for Jo to see the counsellors again. By this time, the family had done more research and had found out that her mum's paternal aunts had all either had bowel or cervical cancer; information which they also gave to the cancer geneticists. Jo was then told that her mum's cancer was now 90 per cent certain to be genetic, and she was offered the BRCA1 and 2 test. Jo asked what would happen if the test came back negative, and was told this would not mean she would be excluded from preventive surgery or screening due to the limitations of the test. She would still be eligible for all these options, based on her family history alone.

In April 2010, the results came back negative, which merely means the fault had not been found. At that time, the Oxford Genetics clinic suggested Jo consult a breast surgeon, although they were unsure whether a surgeon would see her. A letter was written to Reading breast team who, after chasing them up, informed Jo they would *not* perform surgery or even meet to discuss the options. They also said they would no longer see Jo for MRIs as she had moved from the area. Her new area did not offer this screening. Jo really did not know which way to move.

I sent all Jo's details to Professor Evans, our advisor. Here is Jo's letter to me, following on from this:

In under 24 hours, the Helpline achieved more for me than the health service had in the past three years. Before contacting the Helpline I had literally reached a brick wall with the NHS. Nobody seemed to understand about genetics, even though I had done enough of my own research to know that my risk of developing breast cancer was high enough to qualify for risk-reducing surgery. After being refused surgery from my hospital, I didn't know what to do. I still don't know what I would have done if it wasn't for the Helpline. Not only did it provide support through an understanding by Wendy of the issues and emotions I was feeling, but it also gave practical support. In under 24 hours Wendy had sent my details to Prof Evans and he agreed to see me. Within three months I was seeing the surgeon, something I hadn't managed in over three years of trying. I am eternally grateful to the Helpline and the invaluable and unique service it provides.

Jo had her surgery at the Royal Marsden Hospital. She was bright and chirpy almost immediately afterwards, sending me text messages and updating me on how she was feeling. This was a great pleasure for me, and gave me a wonderful feeling to have been in a position to help.

JULIE

Throughout this whole sordid funding issue, the helpline remained busy. My life had to revolve almost solely around it, and the ongoing battles to maintain it. Sarah Rose, a geneticist in London, asked me if she could pass the number on to one of her patients, Julie, who had recently been found to carry a genetic fault and was not coping too well.

Julie contacted me and, as we chatted, I felt she was drawing on my own pragmatism. I'm always pleased when this happens; it's not an issue of persuasion – one route versus another – but more one of empowerment. Julie's family history was not good. In fact, it was awful, similar to my own. She told me over the days we spoke of the sheer bad luck with which this family has been affected.

The gene had been passed on to Julie by her father, whose mother and sister had both died from ovarian cancer. They had died in their fifties, as Julie said, when they should have been able to relax and enjoy life; watch grandchildren grow up, maybe take a few well-deserved holidays. Sadly, none of this happened for

them. Their vicious ovarian cancer could not be successfully overcome.

Julie's cousin Debbie had developed breast cancer at
age 29, when she had young children. Debbie had been
put on Tamoxifen treatment for 11 years, and was
taken off it at age 40. Julie, still clearly strongly affected
by her memories, told me just what a beautiful girl
Debbie was, both in looks and personality. During
Debbie's treatment, which she stoically accepted,
Debbie once said to Julie, 'The trouble is, Julie, you are
just a number.' Very soon after coming off the Tamoxifen
treatment, Debbie was diagnosed with a terminal
spread from the breast cancer. It had metastasised
throughout her body, and she was dying. She told Julie
that the hardest thing she had ever had to do was to
tell her children she was dying.

Debbie stayed at home and Julie spoke with her the
day before she died. How Julie described this to me
had both of us in tears. She said that Debbie was barely
audible, her breathing had become laboured, struggling to keep her alive. Debbie had been afraid of death,
and was reassured that most people just slip away in
their sleep. However, Julie said that far from dying in
her sleep, Debbie was fully conscious. She even tried to
escape. She had attempted to get to the front door –
probably as a way to try to run from the clutches of
death. The picture Julie conjured up for me was poign-
ant beyond belief.

Julie's cousin Carol had also suffered a long-
protracted battle with the disease. It returned in one
shape or another four times over a 22-year period from
the time she was 37 until her death at age 59. Carol,
although initially sceptical of Julie's proposals to have
elective surgery, came to understand this decision

shortly before her own untimely death. As Julie says, Carol was a force to be reckoned with. She was affectionately known as a 'real character'. The love of her family kept her going. She had kept saying to Julie, 'What on earth do you want to mutilate your body for?' Yet Julie felt it was sensible to undergo surgery before this ghastly disease could get a grip. What upset Julie more than anything was that *none* of the women in her family ever had that choice. The BRCA gene had been doggedly passing from generation to generation, leaving no women in her family unaffected by it.

Over the next few months I heard from Julie in fits and starts. She knew I was there if she wanted me, but for the time being I think she was putting things into perspective. Julie's husband, Michael, was trying to be strong, but here was something he could not fix for her. They had recently moved to Norfolk, so Julie was away from her family and friends when she heard that she too had inherited the gene.

At Julie's request, we arranged a visit, which was thwarted by the snow. I liked Julie enormously, and she became a great friend. She knew of the skydive, and the other funding issues, and took it upon herself to visit her MP, Norman Lamb. So impassioned was Julie over the cause that Mr Lamb wrote an excellent letter to the Secretary of State for Health, Andrew Lansley, pleading the case for sensible central funding. Many patients did exactly the same; letters from MPs up and down the country flew to Andrew Lansley's office.

By the time Julie met us, she had decided for herself the route to take. Her surgeon had said to her, 'Julie, you have the BRCA gene. It's not if, it's when.' Although probably not 100 per cent accurate, the fact that approximately 85 out of every 100 women with this fault *will* develop breast cancer in their lifetime, does make his statement 'odds on' as being correct.

As her operation date neared, Julie felt the need to get her head round the whole thing. We arranged to meet at my home. I love having people over as friends and, as usual, we got on so well. Becky came over for lunch and performed her customary routine of allowing fine scrutiny, prodding, poking, and generally any form of examination of her breasts that people wished. Julie was amazed at their appearance. Amazed and encouraged.

Julie's surgery was carried out by Elaine Sassoon, a very well-known and respected surgeon in Norfolk. She now says it was the best decision she ever made and has absolutely no regrets whatsoever. Sadly, her cousin, Carol's daughter, has just been diagnosed with the BRCA gene at age 39, and Carol's 29-year-old niece has developed breast cancer. She has a two-year-old child. And so the gene continues, but Julie has now given it as good a shot as she can. She is herself hoping to train to work on the helpline and join the team.

HEREDITARY BREAST CANCER
AWARENESS WEEK 2010

As the Awareness Week approached, individual press releases were compiled for each local newspaper, each one citing the preposterous excuse their own PCT had given to refuse our funding. All local radio stations were contacted, as well as TV and national media. It was a monster task, but one Becky and I took on between us with some fervour. In the end we had booked in 16 radio interviews for the first day. Press releases flew out to every local paper we could find. The whole episode was insane!

I began the day at six a.m., installed in a studio at Radio Sheffield and talking to most local radios 'down the line', as it's known, at five-minute intervals. Some of the skydivers went to different radio stations, and somehow at local level we covered the whole country. I had by this time written up the excuses given by the PCTs for not funding this tiny £422; it read more like a comedy script than a set of responsible bodies in charge of £100 billion of *our* healthcare money.

After a full day of these interviews, I dashed down to Bakewell to the post office to catch the post. As I reached the front of the queue, my mobile phone rang. I had diverted the Helpline to it so this was nothing out of the ordinary. What was out of the ordinary, though, was that it was Radio Hampshire, ringing to do an interview. Oh heck, I must have forgotten about that one. I was on air in seconds. I abandoned all my belongings at the counter and dashed around the busy shop, trying to find a quieter place from which to talk about hereditary breast cancer and naughty PCTs. Not easy. I finally plumped for the photo booth, but I can't say I was very focused on that interview. Anyone from Hampshire who recalls an incoherent Drivetime interview – I apologise. Profusely.

On the morning of the skydive, we picked everyone up in the coach and I was overwhelmed by the palpable fear some were clearly experiencing. Everyone was in their own private little terrified world. Pale faces stared blankly ahead. Every single person there was silently enacting all the likely scenarios of failed or faulty parachutes, instructors passing out before pulling the cord, and every other imaginable deadly occurrence. Many of them, like Becky and Paula, were petrified even of flying, let alone jumping from 13,500 feet!

As we pulled closer to the airfield, the coach driver asked over the microphone, 'This is your last chance, anyone want to get out here?' A ripple of nervous laughter echoed round the coach, which served to break the ice somewhat.

We pulled into the car park and unloaded the gazebo. We were now the proud owners of a quantity of various stock items – T-shirts, sweatshirts and other various merchandise – all showing the helpline logo (some even in diamanté!) to help give us a presence at the various county shows and rallies we were attending.

Everyone busied themselves setting up, the sun was shining, and the instructors were totally brilliant. They had the group rolling with laughter at the short training course, and the tension was broken. Everyone donned their PCT T-shirt, and photos were duly taken. It really was the most amazing day. I chatted to them all, expressing my gratitude and respect for their incredible bravery, and their success in getting their sponsorship money.

A small, rather basic plane flew three or four people at a time for their 'jump'. Once aboard, they were carefully strapped to their allotted instructor – having already undergone instructions as to what to do when they landed.

I sat at a picnic table and, as each skydiver returned to earth, I asked them to give me all their thoughts, how they felt, and so on. Gary, our wonderful cameraman, took a great deal of film, asking the same thing of everyone, both before and after the jump. One or two telling quotes were that they wanted to help because the PCTs weren't doing their bit. The whole day had a really marvellous feel about it. So warm and happy, generous and caring. I couldn't help thinking just how far this had come on in the past three months. From being a lone warrior, I now had an army to myself! Gary set the whole film to the song 'Woman on a Mission'. How appropriate. We gave everyone a small glass trophy as a keepsake, with the motto, 'You cannot know what a difference you have made.'

Everyone who jumped was just so ecstatic after the event. It must have been quite a spectacle to see, 'Jumping for SOUTHAMPTON', or whichever of the PCTs they had taken on, written on all the T-shirts. Every skydiver had raised sponsorship money of at least £500. The cost of the jump and the other incidentals totalled around £250, so we knew we were on to a winner.

Paula had raised the most money. She had been sponsored by so many great connections from the Chatsworth Estate and the Duke of Devonshire's family, that her total was over £2,000. We gave her three PCTs to 'jump' for. Shortly before the skydive, I had been informed that Newcastle Northumberland and North of Tyne, previously good payers, had refused to pay for 2010/2011. The original commissioner, who had a very high opinion of the helpline, was now on maternity leave and the new commissioner did not want to pay for the service. This left me really querying the reasoning behind everything. How could funding decisions depend on a commissioner's pregnancy? Because that is what it amounted to.

I had been invited to give a talk at a group support meeting in the Centre for Life, Newcastle, to all the BRCA faulty gene carriers. At the end of the session, one of the ladies stood up. She said that after her diagnosis of carrying one of these gene faults she had come to rely upon the website and its service. She stated how important it had been for her, how easy the fact sheet was to read, and finally said, 'We should all be given this number when we get our genetic test results.' The entire room agreed with her. The geneticists witnessed this.

I wrote to the commissioners and the North England Cancer Network Director, Roy McLachlan, telling them all of this. I received no further communication whatsoever. The really sensible commissioner in Gateshead told me that he was, quite frankly, amazed by his colleagues. He had himself offered to do the skydive. I was struggling with which PCTs to get him to 'jump' for. It appealed to my sense of humour to have a Director of Commissioning for a PCT jumping to cover for a non-paying colleague! He couldn't jump for his own as he had already paid. It would take some explaining, that's for sure, and was probably not easy for him either.

Of course, as expected, this was now total war. The local papers picked it up with a vengeance. I was told that it had pressed panic buttons in the cancer networks up and down the country. Statements were requested from these PCTs and cancer networks by radio stations and newspapers as to why they did not pay this very small amount for a service that came so highly recommended by NICE. It was obviously much needed and used.

I received a copy of an email from a director of one of the cancer networks, the quangos that advise the PCTs. I laughed my head off over her comments: 'My PCTs have capitulated under the weight of MP letters, haranguing from the media and skydiving cancer patients.'

What was upsetting, though, was that initially this woman had met me a year or so before at the NOWGEN training course I lectured at. She had vowed to help me with the funding issues in London, which she did. Now she had moved 'networks' and was involved with her colleagues in the campaign against me that was being waged up and down the country. What a war I had started, all over £422. I could have understood it if the reason for difficult decisions and so on could be substantiated, but looking into the PCT Annual Reports showed such colossal waste, huge salaries paid and £108 million in management cost discrepancies. In the face of all this, my £422 was nothing. In addition to this, the Department of Health had commissioned a review of services for hereditary breast cancer and concluded this was the *only* service available and was, therefore, essential.

In 2006, the NICE Guideline Committee discussed the matter of consistent information for patients. The patient booklet clearly stated that the patient should receive Standard Written Information at their initial GP consultation, whether they were being referred or not. No one had co-ordinated this, so it still wasn't happening. I took it on myself, working with a committee of top professionals, to produce these two simple sheets. We had the sheets 'peer reviewed' and approved through all the relevant committees. The first sheet was entitled, 'You have been referred for genetic counselling. What happens next?' The other sheet, 'Standard information for patients where no referral deemed necessary', detailed why the patient was not thought to be at sufficiently increased risk, why they had not been referred, and gave advice on breast awareness and further family history research. Both sheets gave the helpline number. As an initiative during Hereditary Breast Cancer Awareness Week, I sent out links to information sheets for GPs to download for their patients. These links were sent to *every* PCT to send out to their GP practices *free of charge*. Amazingly some of the non-paying ones refused to forward the information to their GPs, even though these were written by the Chair of the NICE Guideline Committee and a team of experts, because they hadn't commissioned them! They were free!

During the summer of 2010 it became apparent that the level of work required to keep the national helpline open 24 hours a day was really not sustainable. Running the service every day was becoming a worry for me. I would never ever miss the phone if at all possible, but for how long can someone be on duty every day? I had now been on hand for 14 years, and it was necessary to train others. It was vital for the knowledge I had amassed over the years to be more widely known. Help is needed for the three per cent of the female population for whom we are to be the sole support. Leaflets need posting, need to be available everywhere. Each woman unaware of her risk was a potential death. How could I not worry that we weren't doing enough?

I must train others to help. From within the over 5000-strong database, we recruited 22 people to train to work on the helpline. All I have left to do now is batter the doors down for funding. It is one thing being unable to pay yourself – quite another not to pay others. So far we have survived on the contributions from those PCTs who do pay, together with periodic injections of money from the various fundraising events. Those funds were intended to finance the training and awareness ventures, not cover the day-to-day running costs. I have just managed. I suppose I am a bit gung-ho. Nothing bar total poverty would stop me here, but of course this lack of finance does not help cover any paid workers. I'm not fazed though. I will continue to fight each day, gathering more and more political, clinical and departmental support, until finally something gives. Hopefully, that something won't be me.

I decided to hold a training weekend for new helpers. We had all attended the one-day course at the NOWGEN Centre in Manchester for the more formal training, tailored to breast care nurses intent on running family history clinics. I was a speaker at this course, and a month later we held the more informal residential weekend. I had no idea how this would work. For a start, I had to write the training manual – this had never been done before as we are still the only helpline in the world for this group of people. The training weekend was fantastic. We were fortunate to have the opportunity to use Manor Court, a beautiful group of holiday cottages in Over Haddon. It worked splendidly; everyone mucked in to get the place prepared as a group residential weekend. As usual, my talented sister came to the fore with mountains of home-made food to fatten us all up.

The first day was highly emotional. People told their various stories about why they had used the helpline and what value they had personally gained from the resource. Just what had their need been? The weekend more or less ran itself after that. I desperately needed to attract substantial funding so I could employ people full time to work on the helpline. I was lucky enough to have attracted the attention and support of many suitable people who had used the helpline themselves and who were already versed in speaking with others. Lisa Shiers, who initially used the helpline herself some four years earlier, already facilitated a forum for 'at risk' women. She herself was a gene carrier and already understood the necessary boundaries. Lisa had said she would be very interested in getting involved with the helpline. Now was the opportunity.

Having given everyone a chance to share their story and why they used the helpline, we started to pinpoint the main reasons for its need. The feeling of isolation after being told you carried a faulty gene was a common theme throughout. Some felt that others just didn't understand the life-changing decisions that had to be faced. Most felt that although they reached decisions they were comfortable with themselves, well-meaning friends and relatives were always keen to try 'helpfully' to change your mind. We noted these and many other reasons, and I went home to type them up for the next day.

We all got together for a fantastic meal in one of the cottages. The kitchen was bursting at the seams with Diane's goodies, and Tim and Justine from the local golf club delivered our hot food. We pushed three very long tables together and talked until the small hours. This gathering had such a cathartic effect; having the understanding audience gave people a chance to share their experiences, which is essentially much of what is required on the helpline.

The next morning, we all went on a walk in the lovely Lathkildale. I hoped to give everyone a chance to enjoy this weekend too. We were now joined by lead cancer nurse Nicola James, who was also keen to help on the line.

I had written a large paper about procedures and boundaries, hoping to involve people in the understanding of just why any help *must* be non-directional. I think this was well understood and we concluded the weekend by splitting into pairs around the complex and running through the 10 scenarios I had given them; all focused on genuine calls I had received over the years. I was very keen to impress on everyone that it's okay *not* to know all the answers. I always ask people to pop all the questions down in a short email for us to consult with our two tireless, trusty advisors, Gareth and Ros.

At the end of a long weekend, we all agreed how beneficial yet fun it had been. Margaret and Richard were both entranced. Margaret hugged me and cried, saying how this had helped them to actually speak about Suzanne's death. Richard was equally as loving. I was thrilled to have attracted such an eclectic group of people, and felt that no matter who called the helpline in future, there would be several people available who could identify with them. Some weeks earlier, a chance talk at Chatsworth Women's Institute, one of the many WI talks I do around Derbyshire, elicited support from a direction I had not envisaged. Nicola James had been in the audience, and came up to me at the end, telling me how much she enjoyed the talk and would like to help. Her email arrived before I had even managed to get home:

Hi Wendy,

I met you tonight at WI, Chatsworth. I was blown away by your talk. I am the Trust Lead Cancer Nurse for Chesterfield. I am also on the editorial board for a national oncology journal called Cancer Nursing Practice. I am also a nurse consultant for prostate cancer and a couple of years ago won Nursing Standard Innovation in Cancer Award. I am on the NICE guidance group for Cancer of Unknown Primary. I honestly don't mean to bore you with my CV but my point is that I would love to help you in any way I could. I really mean any way, from helping with the helpline to lobbying relevant parties. I have a meeting tomorrow pm with PCT commissioners and am going to tell them what I learnt about tonight under any other business.

Please let me know if I can help you and how. I usually snooze thru WI meetings. I was transfixed by yours.
Nicola James

I wrote back to Nicky immediately, thrilled to get practical support voluntarily from a professional of Nicky's calibre. Of course, the geneticists are all highly supportive. They value and admire the service we provide, but here was someone wanting to be trained to work on the helpline herself, which was invaluable.

Now the trained team are in the wings, waiting to help. But I cannot employ people without knowing they can be paid. The volunteers will be an enormous help, but we need administrative staff and database managers to control all of this. While I am taking the calls and liaising with Gareth myself, I know that everything is being done correctly, but once others are involved you need to have audits to ensure that the advice is sound and well delivered. I am utterly determined that the unblemished reputation of the helpline will be maintained.

HELEN

Helen is one of the largest group, the moderate risk group, that I am constantly concerned with. What is there for them? No clinical support, no genetic test, just the knowledge of a substantially increased risk. Helen appreciates my massive concerns for everyone in this position. Here are a few of her letters to me:

Dear Wendy,
It was lovely to speak to you today, thank you for taking the time to call me, I know you are an incredibly busy lady.

I was delighted to learn of your plans, through your helpline, to provide practical support for women like myself who are classed as at 'moderate' risk of developing breast cancer. This really was music to my ears, I couldn't believe what you were saying. You completely understood my frustrations and understood why I was devastated to be classed as moderate risk.

I have seen a geneticist, who has calculated my lifetime risk of developing breast cancer as 27 per cent, (moderate risk). This is despite my mum dying of breast cancer (when my first born was six weeks old), my maternal nan and great aunt also had it. My mum's sister is currently terminally ill with breast cancer and my mum's cousin was diagnosed last year. Shocking and chilling, isn't it? The fear I feel when I look at my family tree is overwhelming.

Incidentally, despite all these cancers, I was not entitled to a genes test on the NHS, I am one of the lucky ones, I paid privately to have one, I'm not a BRAC1 or 2 carrier, but my geneticist thinks my family has another undiscovered gene in my family that's causing all the cancers.

So I feel completely in no man's land, only moderate risk and not a BRAC carrier. Yet EVERYONE in my family is getting breast cancer.

I was actually devastated when classed as moderate risk, only 3 per cent off high risk. Having looked at the NICE guidelines, it seems that if you are high risk, doors open, more tests are available (MRIs), and you are generally taken more seriously and are looked after. I really wish I was high risk to have access to more support, you are one of the few who understand this.

This has been a life-changing learning curve for me. I was shocked to discover that all there is available to me is an annual mammogram, which obviously I attend. I have read that mammograms in someone my age (36) aren't that effective, but it's all that is on offer so I take it. My geneticist is great, but she only gives me the computer-generated stats, I'm not a statistic, I'm Helen, whose mum died when my little boy was six weeks old. I will never recover from that experience. Harry is now three and a half and I am now blessed with Daisy, six weeks old.

I do attend a local family history clinic annually, when I went last year, I was told I have a greater chance of not developing breast cancer than I do of developing it – that appointment was a waste of time, felt like I was banging my head against a brick wall.

There is no other support for someone like myself, no one to turn to, only your helpline. To hear you are going to try to provide practical and emotional support to the tens of thousands of women in my position is wonderful. It's a support mechanism that is so sadly currently missing but yet so very badly needed. Can I repeat, we are not statistics, but real women with husbands and children who are desperately trying to put a positive spin on our situation, but who sometimes need help.

Thank you for taking the time to read this, please do not hesitate to get in touch Wendy if I can help at all.

Helen xxxx

Helen's letter, of course, is heart-rending. She has kept up to date on our financial position regarding the PCTs and has written several well-worded letters to me. It has been a great support for me to constantly receive these letters. There are numerous of them on our website, posted there for anyone to read and identify with. Many love just to use the website, which normalises this whole faulty gene situation, and puts it in the context of living a normal life.

Just before the Vanessa Feltz show I was invited on to, Helen wrote this next letter to me:

Can't wait to see you on The Vanessa Show, *Wendy. No doubt you will be amazing on the programme as your passion for this cause shines through. Thanks again for all your tireless fighting for us all, we love you to bits, Helen. xxx (Member of Wendy's Army) xxx*

What else could anyone need?

CLAIRE

Claire telephoned the helpline at several stages through her own personal journey. She on many occasions referred to it as her lifeline. During the period of the news being delivered of the Tesco nomination and award, Claire was a constant helpline user. She wanted reading material, people's stories, anything to help her get to grips with this whole situation. In fact, it was due to Claire's desire for reading material that I really put my brain in gear and started writing this book. She readily agreed to travel from Newbury to the Peak District to be filmed by *Tesco Magazine* for the award film they were making about me.

Meeting Claire was delightful. She appreciated every bit of support we were giving to her, endlessly thanked us, and then apologised for thanking us! She has now undergone her first operation, the oophrectomy, the removal of her ovaries. It didn't go as easily as hoped, but nevertheless Claire is well and truly on the mend now. She has set up her own website, *www. claireandthegenie.com*, to which we will put a link from our helpline website, as it is to be a blog on her journey. Claire wrote a section on the helpline for her website, describing her needs and how useful it had all been for her:

When I was first told that I carried the BRCA2 gene muta-tion, it took a few hours for the enormity of my situation to dawn on me and when it did, I picked up the phone to Wendy. Wendy Watson founded the National Hereditary Breast Cancer Helpline over ten years ago. Within minutes of speaking to her my terror began to subside – I wasn't alone.

Wendy and the team, which includes her daughter Becky, are on the other end of this phone 24 hours a day to listen and give advice to people just like me. Wendy was the first person to have a preventative mastectomy and Becky was the youngest – at just 24. This family have not only managed to overcome their own fears but they have put so much back into helping other people with hereditary cancer and also supporting those at risk.

The team at the helpline can put you in touch with other people who are in the same situation – providing telephone numbers so you can talk to somebody who has been through it. I have spoken to numerous girls who have either had their operations or who are at the same stage as I am. It has been great to compare stories and to comfort each other, each conversation being intermittently inter-rupted with 'I know what you mean.'

I first picked up the phone to the helpline when I was waiting for my genetic test results. The genetic team had given me a flyer with the helpline number and I rang it almost immediately. I then sent endless emails which allowed me to off-load the fear without burdening my husband. In the middle of the night I would rant about how scared I was and how I could think of nothing else.

Wendy would calmly reply or ring me the next day, just checking I was OK.

Wendy also sent me two brilliant DVDs which I would also recommend watching. Both are available through the helpline website and describe Wendy and Becky's journeys from discovering they have the gene to after their operations. I found both their stories inspiring and it gave me huge comfort to actually see another girl go through the same experience and remain so positive.

Ironically this helpline has very little funding and in the future I am hoping to get involved in fundraising, expanding the helpline and setting up local support groups. It has helped me to 'stay on track' and remain positive. My story is one of many so please contact the helpline by phone or email if you feel they can help you – or indeed if you think you can help them!

Claire is clearly yet another who has found support – and has been empowered to take control of her own destiny, because this is what it's all about. We all need to take control of our own health. It is just not enough to pass the responsibility on to the GP who, learned as he or she may be, cannot possibly know everything about us and be a mindreader too. This is where we are at with the helpline. Our mission statement is 'Educating the World' but in the most positive manner possible. Make people aware of all the options that are currently available then ensure they receive full support, no matter what their choice.

I have recently completed a piece of research into the cost benefits of this surgery in 'identified gene carriers'. It demonstrates that for every 100 women who undergo risk-reducing surgery, over 40 lives are saved and at least £1,880,000. This has been submitted by a patient to

BUPA resulting in agreement to fund their surgery privately; thus creating an invaluable precedent.

Luckily, this *Tesco Magazine* Award news has now prompted some action. Ministers are requesting meetings with me. The Department of Health have said they are concerned. Bob Park from North East London Cancer Network is working hard for me. Now I have to write back to all the 110 PCTs who have so far refused to pay this year and re-submit the tiny invoice for £422. Their curt refusals to pay, though, are at least offset by others who are helping in this war. Because that is just what it is – but I am constantly supported by the patients and clinicians who will not let this go.

I feel even more certain that, somehow or other, I will get the necessary funding to continue and to grow. My optimism for the future refuses to give up now. So many patients, now friends whom I have got to know so well, are declaring the most glorious things about both myself and this service. 740 lives saved in England alone! Of course I *must* fight on!

And I will.

TESCO MAGAZINE MUM OF THE YEAR AWARDS

Waldorf Hotel, 27 February 2011

And so I received a call from Lisa at *Tesco Magazine*. The first call came totally out of the blue, and I was actually talking to somebody on the helpline at the time. I asked if it would be all right for me to call back, and assumed there was to be a feature on breast cancer and they wanted a few statistics or to include the helpline number. Lisa said that was fine, she would call back shortly.

When she did, what she told me was unbelievable. Becky had written and nominated me for the *Tesco Magazine* Mum of the Year Award – and I had got down to the final 18. This was out of a total of over 4,000 letters. I was thrilled to have got this far!

I rang Becky straight away, dreading her not answering, but she was there. When I told her I was down to the final 18 she squealed with delight.

'Mum, go on the website and look it up. It's a fantastic award ceremony.' And so I did. But I didn't want to get to know too much in case I was disappointed. The final 18 was good enough really, I told myself!

Lisa and Debbie arranged they would call back and

arrange a trip to interview me before the final selections. At this point Becky was beside herself with excitement.

'Please, Mum, don't go on about PCTs, will you?'

I suppose I had to admit that I had now got such a one-track mind over this interminable fight for survival. Of course I promised I wouldn't and I knew that the story is so long with its many diversions, I would be unlikely to reach that point quickly.

Debbie and Lisa arrived at my home one Monday. They were lovely people and I warmed to them both straight away. I had prepared some lunch for them – not to my sister's standard, but hopefully appetising – and we all sat in my living room. We talked and talked and talked. Eventually they told me the time of their train back, so I quickly force-fed them and drove them to the railway station in Chesterfield. Then the waiting began. How had my interview gone, I wondered? All I could do was tell my story. Debbie said they would call me either way in around 10 days.

After two weeks, when I thought that the silence was not a good sign, I suddenly received a call while I was in the bank. Debbie. She asked if I could talk. I explained I was in the bank so she said she would call back in 10 minutes or so. A further hour elapsed, no call.

That's it, I thought.

Eventually the call came.

Debbie started off with, 'Well, I did tell you we would let you know either way.' My heart sank. Here was the big let-down, probably with reassuring words about stiff opposition and so forth. This lasted less than a second because, after a tiny pause, Debbie said, 'And I'm pleased to tell you that you are one of our eight winners.'

She then went on to explain the even more exciting

fact that I was the overall winner. Oh my goodness! I became a total incomprehensible wreck after that. I had no idea what else I was told, except that it must not get out yet. I could tell just close family and that was about it. How on earth you are supposed to keep that news to yourself I have no idea. Chris and Becky were over the moon, as were Dad and Olive. And Diane. And my very closest friends.

Becky actually screamed when I phoned her. All she could say was, 'NO! No way!!! No way!!!'

How marvellous to have this sort of relationship with your daughter and how gratifying to realise just how proud she was of me.

The run-up to the awards seemed a long way off, but the time passed in a whirlwind of calls from stylists, photographers, production companies making the short film about our stories, and the PR company. Everyone was so kind and encouraging.

Andy Burnham invited me to see him. He was keen to help with my funding issues and so thrilled at my award. He was eager to meet me face to face and wanted to tell me just how important he felt the helpline was. He agreed to be filmed for the award ceremony and explain just what I and the helpline had meant to him. His transcript is an unbelievable testimonial from a former Minister of Health.

The excitement built even further. Becky and I headed for the train station, loaded with dresses and shoes and the thousand or so other necessary items women need for a two-day stay in London. The generosity of Tesco with my dress and all the matching accessories for the day was brilliant. Jo, the top stylist employed by Tesco, tried to turn us ordinary mums into glamour pusses for

the occasion. And she succeeded – we all looked absolutely wonderful.

As we arrived at the Waldorf Hotel, the *Tesco Magazine*
Mum of the Year team, headed by Debbie Chernin,
were there to greet us. Our rooms were filled with gifts,
champagne, flowers, chocolates . . . and a very precise
timetable of events.

The schedule for the big day was really comical:
breakfast delivered to the room at seven a.m.; at eight
a.m. the hairdresser, make-up artist and stylists would
all arrive; a film crew would turn up just after nine to
film the preparation process. We were told there were
80 people working behind the scenes to make this
event happen, and I'm firmly convinced that every
single one of them was in my room at half past nine. So
funny – and I hadn't even made the bed. Becky had
even managed to get fake tan all over her crisp white
Egyptian-cotton bed sheets!

People wondered if I had breast prostheses in for the
event. I didn't. As I've already recounted, I used to have
endless mishaps with these things, which led to my
wearing them only occasionally. Most of the time I
would wear nothing and, amazingly, people didn't
really notice. Perhaps they thought I was exceptionally
flat-chested, or didn't notice at all. Who cares. So long
as I feel I look all right, that's the main thing. To be
honest, I never think about it at all these days.

The gorgeous Palm Court Room at the Waldorf was
just perfect for the occasion. Not too large, but very
light and airy with a colour scheme which perfectly
matched the gold and white theme of the *Tesco Magazine*
Mum of the Year logo. We watched as the room was
transformed. It was filled with flowers, and the lovely

balustrade gallery led beautifully onto the stage area. We had a further rehearsal, followed by photo shoots, and at one p.m. the walk along the red carpet. Good gracious – I had never in my life expected something like this to happen. Paparazzi were all eagerly waiting to snap the celebrities lined up to attend the event, probably grudgingly as we were not yet well known, but it was still an amazing experience. A very distinguished gentleman looking rather like Lord Snowdon took my photograph and asked me my name. He was from *OK!* magazine. Gosh! Then it was time to return to our special area to wait for our announcement and the 'walk in' to the heady music chosen to herald our entrance.

It was at this point that everything actually did click into place. This whole affair really had been extraordinary from day one! From my discovering the family history to finding a way to cheat it; the nonsensical battles to put things in place for others; newspapers, gene patents, moratoriums on insurance, constant battles with PCTs and others – just to enable a choice for a woman that could possibly save her life. I now saw why the cause was being embraced in such a way. Every one of us mums had our own personal film made about our achievements.

Watching my film, Professor Gareth Evans my stalwart supporter throughout, said it all. He stated how many hundreds of lives had now been saved through my pioneering of an unknown procedure and my battles with the medical profession to change their views. He spoke of my persistence in getting the media to accept – and report – this as a sensible option, not a bizarre occurrence. They showed pictures of the European Parliament, and of headlines in all the broadsheets about ordinary Wendy Watson, taking on the might of the European Parliament. And then there was fighting a £30million lobby and the pharmaceutical industry, the further challenges of gene patent applications, and of the insurance industry in their rights to ask for genetic test results. And now the endless fights with the Primary Care Trusts to keep the service going. We watched and listened to the emotional and heartfelt thanks of Claire, who sat talking to camera, tearfully grateful for the continuous support she was receiving.

Yes, I suppose it *is* all extraordinary. The smiles and laughs echo around the room as I explain that Wendy Watson versus Myriad Genetics is in the syllabus at Princeton University, and giggling on the film and saying, 'How ridiculous is that?' I don't suppose that's too ordinary either.

Two standing ovations are completely awesome. Just one would have been incredible.

It all seemed a long way from watching my mum and my grandma grow ill and die from their cancers, then living under the shadow myself of this most horrific disease, to helping others find suitable help for themselves. Despite being no medical expert, I recognised and understood the importance of women being able to receive the individual help each and every one of them needed. And then there was the necessity to change perceptions. How gratifying that a procedure I had to invent for myself, which was viewed either as bizarre, or as extreme overreaction, is now recommended by NICE. The fact that I have been asked to talk in so many countries and challenged as to my own sanity, has just been rewarded in the most fulfilling way. The honour of becoming *Tesco Magazine* Mum of

ABOUT THE HELPLINE

The Helpline is open 24 hours every day 01629 813000.

Email canhelp@btopenworld.com

Website www.breastcancergenetics.co.uk

Facebook: National Hereditary Breast Cancer Helpline. Since writing this book we now have local support groups around the country.

Details available on our website.

Whilst the helpline is non-directional, and does not promote one course of action over another, we now have a gallery of photographs on our website showing the different surgical options and results. We also have an easy, patient friendly, fact sheet which can be downloaded. We hope you enjoy our website. It is full of uplifting stories and testimonials. Please join us in our events. We would love to see you!